Medical Emergencies Guide for Dental Auxiliaries

FIFTH EDITION

Medical Emergencies Guide for Dental Auxiliaries

FIFTH EDITION

Melissa Damatta, MSDH, RDH, CDA/
Vaishali Singhal, DMD, Ph.D., MS/Debra Jennings, DMD

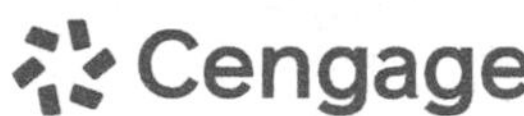

Australia • Brazil • Canada • Mexico • Singapore • United Kingdom • United States

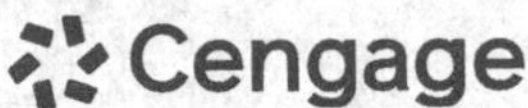

***Medical Emergencies Guide for Dental Auxiliaries*, Fifth Edition**
Melissa Damatta, Vaishali Singhal, Debra Jennings

SVP, Higher Education & Skills Product: Erin Joyner

Product Director: Jason Fremder

Product Manager: Lauren Whalen

Product Assistant: Dallas Wilkes

Content Manager: Sharib Asrar, MPS

Digital Delivery Lead: David O'Connor

Director, Product Marketing: Neena Bali

Marketing Manager: Courtney Cozzy

IP Analyst: Ashley Maynard

IP Project Manager: Kelli Besse

Production Service: MPS Limited

Designer: Chris Doughman

Cover Image Source: saile/ShutterStock.com

Library of Congress Control Number: 2021903642

ISBN: 978-0-357-45692-7

Cengage
200 Pier 4 Boulevard
Boston, MA 02210
USA

Cengage is a leading provider of customized learning solutions with employees residing in nearly 40 different countries and sales in more than 125 countries around the world. Find your local representative at **www.cengage.com.**

To learn more about Cengage platforms and services, register or access your online learning solution, or purchase materials for your course, visit **www.cengage.com.**

Notice to the Reader

Publisher does not warrant or guarantee any of the products described herein or perform any independent analysis in connection with any of the product information contained herein. Publisher does not assume, and expressly disclaims, any obligation to obtain and include information other than that provided to it by the manufacturer. The reader is expressly warned to consider and adopt all safety precautions that might be indicated by the activities described herein and to avoid all potential hazards. By following the instructions contained herein, the reader willingly assumes all risks in connection with such instructions. The publisher makes no representations or warranties of any kind, including but not limited to, the warranties of fitness for particular purpose or merchantability, nor are any such representations implied with respect to the material set forth herein, and the publisher takes no responsibility with respect to such material. The publisher shall not be liable for any special, consequential, or exemplary damages resulting, in whole or part, from the readers' use of, or reliance upon, this material.

Printed in the United States of America
Print Number: 02 Print Year: 2022

Contents

Preface

Introduction

Medical emergencies can and do occur within the dental office environment. A large percentage of these emergencies can be prevented or at least better treated if all the members of the dental team are more knowledgeable in the prevention and management of medical emergency situations.

The *Medical Emergencies Guide for Dental Auxiliaries* is designed to provide dental auxiliary students with the basic skills and knowledge necessary to function effectively as a member of the dental team. This text is also an effective refresher tool for dental auxiliaries who are already working in dentistry. The format of this textbook will help the reader master new information and will simplify review of previously learned materials.

Why We Wrote This Text

This text contains basic information in a format that allows the educator to use the content as written or increase the knowledge base as appropriate for the level of the students.

Chapter Organization

The fifth edition of *Medical Emergencies Guide for the Dental Auxiliary* has been updated to represent up-to-date information regarding the most common medical emergencies encountered in the dental office. The layout and order are a result of listening to our customers and designing a structure that makes sense to those who use this text on a regular basis. Creating sections and grouping chapters in a logical framework is what makes this textbook successful.

This edition of the textbook is organized into six sections containing a total of 14 chapters. The sections are arranged by type of emergency for easier reference and a more reader-friendly approach to various emergencies that can occur in a dental practice. For example, Section III: Respiratory Distress Emergencies contains chapters on respiratory emergencies that can happen in the dental setting. This organization will help the dental auxiliary student learn about related emergencies and the similarities and differences in how to handle them.

Because the guidelines for Cardiopulmonary Resuscitation (CPR) can change at any time, we found it best to remove the chapter on CPR to keep the textbook as up to date as possible. In addition, the dental auxiliary should be trained and certified in Basic Life Support, making the chapter an unnecessary addition.

The organization of this fifth edition is designed to ensure that those pursuing careers as dental professionals will have all the necessary skills and information to be prepared to effectively handle a medical emergency in the dental office with confidence.

Features

The fifth edition contains the following chapter elements:

Key Terms: Important terms are listed alphabetically at the beginning of each chapter and found in the Glossary at the end of the textbook.

Learning Outcomes: At the beginning of each chapter, these objectives address the concepts the reader should understand, and they allow immediate feedback on comprehension.

Test Your Knowledge: Short-answer questions are found throughout the chapters after core concepts have been introduced. These exercises are included to challenge the reader's knowledge and application of the material presented and to facilitate problem solving.

Emergency Basics: These boxed features, which facilitate understanding of important emergency protocols, warning signs and symptoms of an impending emergency, and more are presented succinctly for quick and easy reference.

Summary: Each chapter includes a summary section that synthesizes chapter content covered and highlights main points.

Review Questions: Each chapter includes multiple-choice and true/false questions to add another element of challenge for the reader, and to allow readers to double-check their progress and identify areas where further study is necessary.

Medical Emergency!: Engaging and thought-provoking case studies are located at the end of each chapter, after the review questions. These exercises inspire critical thinking and application of the material learned in the chapter to real-life emergency situations like those readers may face in the professional setting.

Glossary: The end of the textbook contains a complete listing of all key terms and their definitions for a quick and handy reference.

References: Found at the end of the textbook, this material provides students and instructors with resources that may be utilized for further inquiry.

New to the Fifth Edition

- Each chapter is revamped to include higher order of learning objectives to promote critical thinking.
- A new updated title better represents the content of the textbook.
- Chapter 1: Office Preparation, the roles and responsibilities during an emergency situation were merged to be more organized in one list.

- Chapter 2: Medical History, example in a digital format has been added to address the increasing use of dental technology software.
- The previous Chapter 12 was removed due to dental auxiliaries being certified in BLS/CPR.
- Chapter 13: (old Chapter 14), removed dental emergencies because this topic is separate from medical emergencies.
- The Test Your Knowledge feature has been updated to reinforce important concepts and to add another critical-thinking component to the chapters.
- In the Medical Emergency sections, case studies have been updated to reflect possible situations that a dental auxiliary may face. Each case is tailored to the type of emergency that is the focus of the chapter.
- Key Terms, Learning Outcomes, and Review Questions all have been enhanced and updated with the chapter content changes to provide accurate and relevant study components. Key terms have been removed from the margin to allow more room for content.
- Many new figures, tables, and color photographs provide visual illustrations of the content to help further comprehension of important procedures and equipment used during medical emergencies.
- A larger and darker font was used for readability.

Accompanying Teaching and Learning Resources

Spend less time planning and more time teaching with Delmar Cengage Learning's Instructor Resources to Accompany the *Emergency Guide for Dental Auxiliaries, fifth edition.* All Instructor Resources can be accessed by going to www.cengagebrain.com and creating a unique user log-in. The password-protected Instructor Resources include the following:

Online Instructor's Manual

An Instructor Manual accompanies this book. It includes answers to the Test Your Knowledge and Review Questions, as well as additional case studies and exercises for access at any time.

PowerPoint® Lecture Slides

These vibrant, customizable Microsoft® PowerPoint lecture slides for each chapter assist you with your lecture by providing concept coverage using images, figures, and tables directly from the textbook!

Cengage Learning Testing Powered by Cognero

Cengage Learning Testing Powered by Cognero is a flexible online system that allows you to author, edit, and manage test bank content from multiple Cengage Learning solutions; create multiple test versions in an instant; and deliver tests from your LMS, your classroom, or wherever you want.

About the Authors

Melissa Damatta began her career as a dental assistant at a young age. Her love of dentistry motivated her to return to school and pursue dental hygiene. Upon graduation, she immediately returned to school to pursue her second love: education. She began her education career at Rutgers School of Health Professions as an adjunct in the department of Allied Dental Education, where she taught both clinical and didactic courses. During that time she sought out her Certified Dental Assistant (CDA) certification. Melissa went on to teach in the dental hygiene program for Burlington County College in New Jersey. Currently, Ms. Damatta is an associate professor for the dental hygiene program at Community College of Philadelphia, where she serves as clinic coordinator for second-year students and teaches radiology and a preclinical course to first-year students. She has practiced dental hygiene for 18 years, with experiences in periodontal, pediatric, and general dentistry. A former president of Central New Jersey Dental Hygiene Association (CNDHA), she holds memberships in the American Dental Hygiene Association (ADHA) and the American Dental Education Association (ADEA). She continues to practice as a clinical dental hygienist for a private practice in New Jersey. Ms. Damatta completed her associate's degree in applied science in dental hygiene from Middlesex County College in New Jersey, her Bachelors of Science in Health Science–education track from The University of Medicine and Dentistry of New Jersey (now part of Rutgers University), and her Masters of Science in Dental Hygiene with an education concentration from the University of Bridgeport in Connecticut.

Vaishali Singhal is an associate professor at Rutgers University's School of Health Professions (SHP) and Rutgers School of Dental Medicine (RSDM) in Newark, New Jersey. Teaching at the university since 2001, she currently serves as program director of the Bachelor of Sciences in Health Sciences Program at SHP as well as course director for Practice Management and Ethics and Jurisprudence for the 3rd and 4th year dental predoctoral dental students at RSDM. At the faculty practice of RSDM, Dr. Singhal specializes in treating patients with serious mental illness. In 2019 she completed her doctoral thesis at SHP, evaluating ways to improve the oral health of patients with serious mental illness. She completed a Master of Science in Health Sciences at Rutgers University in 2011 and received her DMD from the Rutgers School of Dental Medicine in 1993. Her PhD and MS programs included specialized courses in education, which is Dr. Singhal's passion.

Dr. Debra Jennings obtained her DMD degree from the Medical University of South Carolina (MUSC) in Charleston, South Carolina, during the class of 1990. With a 21-year experience at Trident Technical College, she taught in the Dental Hygiene and Expanded Duty Dental Assistant programs. During this time she also taught a clinical course to the first-year dental students at MUSC to enhance their knowledge of four-handed dentistry. Before attending the Medical University of South Carolina, Dr. Jennings earned dual degrees from the University of South Carolina in Archeology/Criminal Justice and Biology/Chemistry. Her more than 30 years of practical experience in the dental field ran the gamut from dental hygiene to dentistry. Dr. Jennings's many years of dental experience placed her in the unique position of being at the pulse of modern teaching and dental practices. In addition to teaching, she authored and edited various texts and articles for the dental community. When not in the academic arena, she volunteered with the Smiles For A Lifetime clinic that services low-income and immigrant populations. She was a South Carolina native and lived in the low county for more than 30 years.

Dedication

To my fiancé, who has believed in me and encouraged me to get where I am today. To my parents who have supported me undeniably. —Melissa Damatta

To my family who has supported me in all of my endeavors. —Vaishali Singhal

Reviewers

LaQuita Caldwell, CDA, RDA, EFDA
Lead Dental Assisting Instructor
Vista College
College Station, TX

Karen Chockley, MA, CDA, MDPMA
Dental Assisting Program Director
Calhoun Community College
Tanner, AL

Sharilyn Eldredge, CDA, COA
Dental Assisting Instructor
Mountainland Technical College
Orem, UT

Calista Kindle, CDA, EFDA
Program Director
Great Lakes Institute of Technology
Erie, PA

Lori Scribner, CDA, PhD
Dental Assisting Program Director
ATA Career Education
Spring Hill, FL

Kim Turner, RDA
Dental Assisting Instructor
Vista College
Fort Smith, AR

Althea Wynn, RDH
Program Director
Ultimate Medical Academy
Clearwater, FL

SECTION ONE

Prevention

This section deals with assessing the patient and the preparation of the office staff.

CHAPTER 1: Office Preparation
CHAPTER 2: Medical History
CHAPTER 3: Vital Signs

CHAPTER 1

Office Preparation

LEARNING OUTCOMES

Upon completion of this chapter, the student will be able to:

- Identify the role of the dental auxiliary during an office emergency
- Explain the importance of an office emergency routine
- Identify the protocol necessary in an emergency situation
- Describe the functions of the auxiliary in relation to the emergency kit
- Differentiate between a manufactured and homemade emergency kit
- Identify the attachments used with an oxygen tank
- Compare and contrast the demand-valve resuscitator with the Ambu bag
- Demonstrate the operation of the oxygen tank

KEY TERMS

adrenal insufficiency
albuterol
allergic
ammonia
ampule
anaphylactic
angina
benzodiazepines
bradycardia
bronchodilators
demand-valve resuscitator
emergency kit
epinephrine
flowmeter
histamine
hypoglycemia
naloxone
nasal cannula
nitroglycerine
opioid
oxygen mask
oxygen tank
regulator
sildenafil
tadalafil
vaporole
vasodilator
verdanafil

INTRODUCTION

Regardless of how much care is taken, not all dental office emergencies can be prevented. Therefore, should an emergency occur, the dental team must be prepared. To be prepared, the members of the dental team should have a well-planned and practiced emergency routine, have available all necessary equipment, and have appropriate emergency numbers posted at all phones. In addition, the entire staff, even those without direct patient contact, should maintain current credentials in basic life support (BLS) or cardiopulmonary resuscitation (CPR). This will allow for rapid recognition of a medical emergency, resulting in more efficient patient management.

OFFICE EMERGENCY ROUTINE

Medical emergencies can be frightening. It is not uncommon to feel a sense of panic or uncertainty if and when an emergency arises. This is why it is important to have a plan of action, assigning specific functions and responsibilities to each team member. The action plan will help team members avoid confusion and prevent a minor medical emergency from becoming a serious or perhaps even a fatal event. Furthermore, it is essential that this plan be practiced so that if and when an emergency occurs, the established protocols and responsibilities can be carried out without hesitation. As these skills are not used often, review of the plan is needed periodically as a refresher. A great way to provide review of the medical emergency action plan is to perform mock emergencies where each team member can practice their role.

Roles and Responsibilities

Every dental office varies in how it designates responsibilities for each person. The following are roles that can be assigned to anyone in the office. The qualifications of each team member will determine how the roles are assigned. Normally, the dental auxiliary would be the person to retrieve the emergency kit and stay with the dentist during the emergency, while the receptionist would be the person to initiate emergency medical service (EMS). The important thing is that each person in the office has been informed about and understands exactly what their responsibilities involve during an emergency situation.

1. *Notify the dentist of the emergency.* The dentist is responsible for everything in their office and must be notified immediately.
2. *Notify EMS.* Have all emergency numbers updated and within easy reach. It is an excellent idea to always keep these numbers posted next to the telephone. When contacting the emergency medical service, report the nature of the emergency and give explicit directions to the office. Here is a checklist for calling in an emergency:
   - State that your need for the rescue unit is an emergency and explain the nature of the emergency, if known.
   - Give the name and age of the injured person.

- Specify the exact location.
- Provide your name and telephone number.
- Stay on the line until the operator instructs you to hang up.

3. *Administer BLS if necessary.* Until a trained professional arrives, it may be necessary for a certified team member to administer BLS. This consists of maintaining an open airway, providing rescue breathing, providing external cardiac compressions, and use of an automated external defibrillator (AED). All auxiliaries should be able certified to provide basic life support if needed.
4. *Monitor vital signs.* Be prepared to take vital signs. This includes blood pressure, temperature, pulse, and respirations. This information is valuable for when the EMS technicians arrive.
5. *Retrieve the emergency kit.* Once an emergency situation is identified, the emergency kit should be brought to the area immediately so that all the available equipment is ready for use. The emergency kit and its contents are discussed in detail later in this chapter.
6. *Retrieve the oxygen tank.* Oxygen is useful in most emergency situations. Have it available even if the cause or type of emergency has yet to be diagnosed.
7. *Retrieve a hard backboard.* CPR cannot be performed effectively on a patient who is in a soft dental chair; therefore, many offices keep available a piece of board that fits in the back of the dental chair underneath the patient. This board should be brought to the patient's operatory and placed near the chair in case CPR becomes necessary. If a backboard is not available, the patient should be placed on the floor of the operatory before CPR is performed.
8. *Assist the dentist by preparing emergency drugs.* Although auxiliaries cannot legally administer drugs, in some states it is legal for them to prepare the drugs for the dentist to administer. Doing so, when allowed, is helpful in situations where several drugs must be given in succession.
9. *Go outside to direct emergency personnel into the office.* This saves valuable time once the rescue unit arrives.
10. *Keep patients in the waiting room calm.* If the emergency is serious, appointments for patients in the waiting room should be rescheduled. Depending on the circumstances, the receptionist can handle this while the patients are in the office or call them later. The patients who are waiting should be informed that there is an emergency situation but should not be given information concerning the patient's identity or the nature of the emergency.

Practice Routine

Once each person in the office understands their responsibilities, the emergency routine must be practiced on a regular basis. How often the routine is practiced is determined by the dentist and should be included in the office manual. An emergency situation should be simulated, with each person performing their assigned functions. A well-prepared staff handles an emergency much more efficiently than one that has not been prepared by performing practice drills.

TEST YOUR KNOWLEDGE

1. What are some roles and responsibilities during a dental office emergency?

2. When initiating EMS, what details should the person who calls for a rescue unit communicate to the emergency medical personnel?

EMERGENCY KIT

There are several types of **emergency kits**. One type that is gaining in popularity is the homemade emergency kit. The homemade kit is usually assembled by the dentist with the help of physicians, pharmacists, and other medical personnel. This type of kit may be stored in a large tackle box, on a set of instrument trays, or in a cart specifically designed by a dental company for that purpose. When the kit is homemade, the dentist knows exactly what is in the kit and is therefore more likely to be able to use each piece of equipment and each drug proficiently. The kit is designed by the dentist to meet their particular needs.

The second type of emergency kit is the manufactured kit (Figure 1-1). These kits, which are available from every major dental supply company, come in a variety of styles. The advantages of the manufactured kit are as follows:

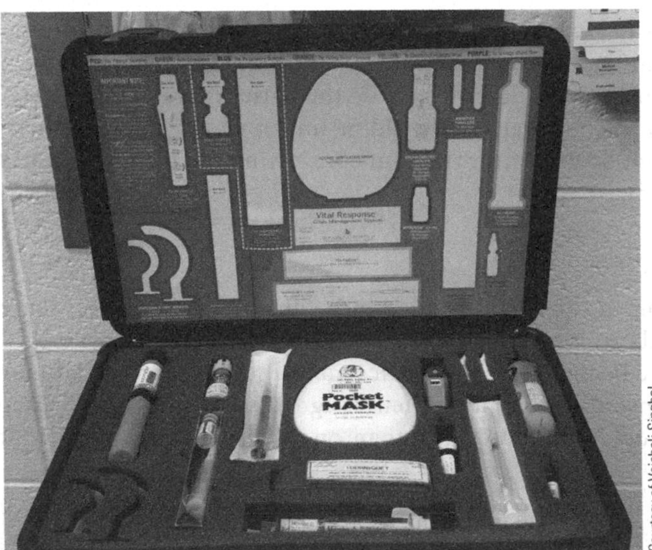

Courtesy of Vaishali Singhal

FIGURE 1-1 Sample emergency kit commonly found in dental settings

- It comes in a carrying case that has compartments specially designed for each item.
- It is designed specifically for dental office emergencies.
- The kit is color coded to match the equipment or drugs with particular types of emergencies.
- Some of these kits are available with prefilled syringes that allow for rapid emergency response.
- The kits often provide for automatic replacement of outdated medications.
- These kits may come with emergency training videos.

The main disadvantage of the manufactured kit is that it can be an elaborate kit containing some equipment and drugs with which the dentist is not completely familiar.

The key to selecting the correct type of emergency kit for any dental office is to make sure it meets the dentist's needs. For example, in an office that is located a great distance from any medical facility, the dentist requires a fairly elaborate emergency kit, whereas a dentist whose office is located across the street from a hospital requires a minimal amount of emergency equipment.

Emergency Kit Contents

Each member of the team should be comfortable and familiar with all of the contents in the emergency kit. In addition to an oxygen delivery system with a positive-pressure capability, at the minimum the following items should be available in the emergency kit. Table 1-1 lists the recommended minimum contents of an emergency kit. Table 1-2 lists additional emergency kit supplies.

TABLE 1-1 Emergency Kit Contents

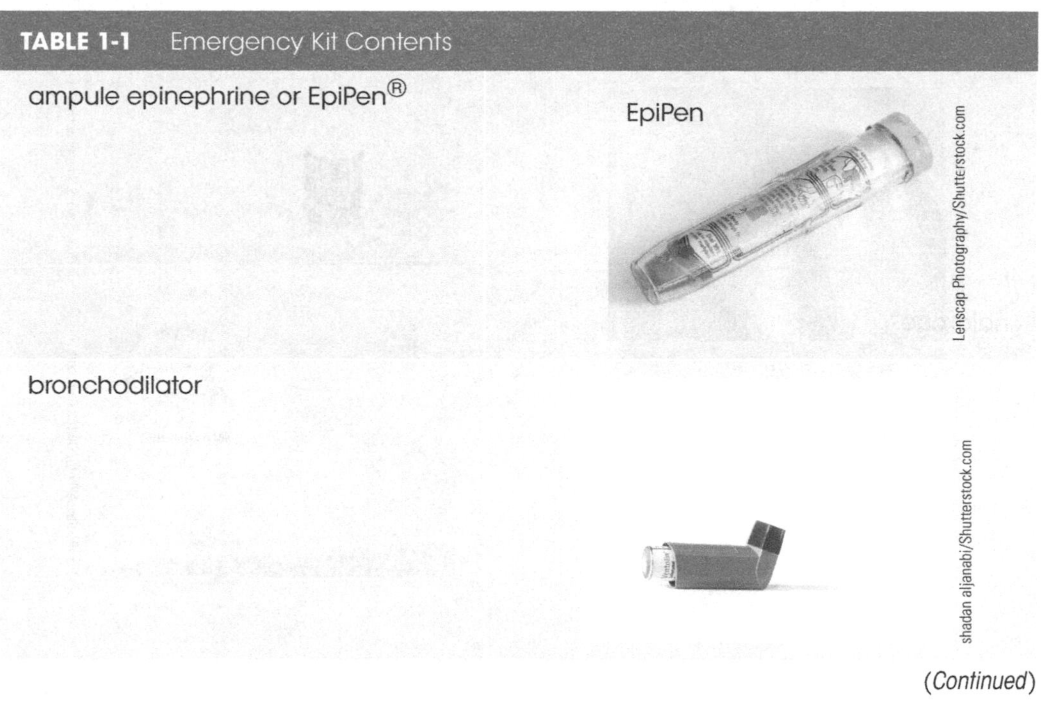

ampule epinephrine or EpiPen®	EpiPen Lenscap Photography/Shutterstock.com
bronchodilator	shadan aljanabi/Shutterstock.com

(Continued)

TABLE 1-1 Emergency Kit Contents

ammonia inhalants	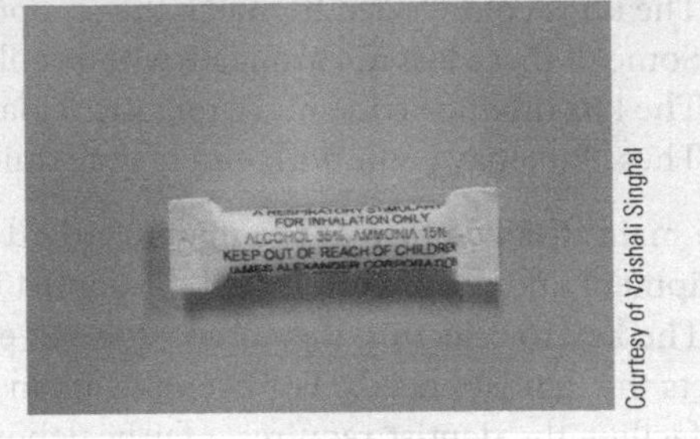 Courtesy of Vaishali Singhal
nitroglycerin tablets or spray	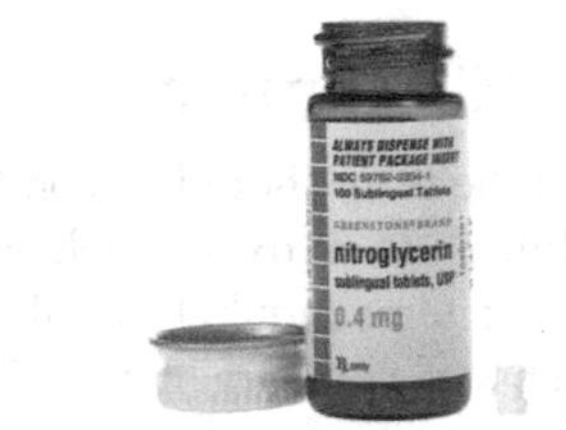 Sheila Fitzgerald/Shutterstock.com
	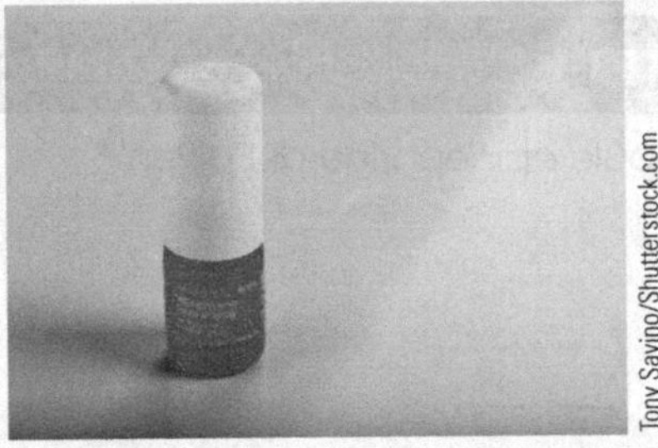 Tony Savino/Shutterstock.com
naloxone	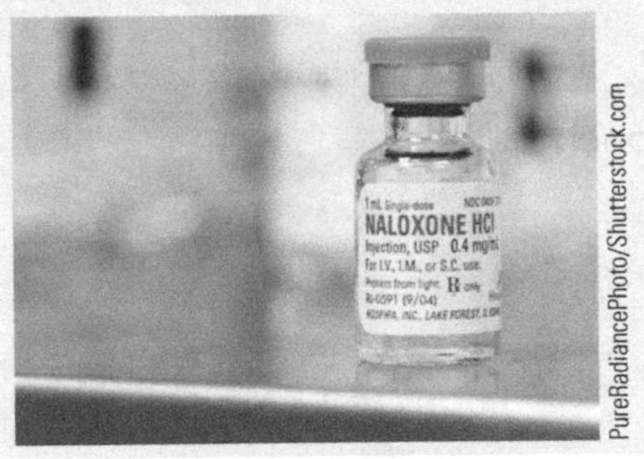 PureRadiancePhoto/Shutterstock.com

TABLE 1-1 Emergency Kit Contents

aspirin	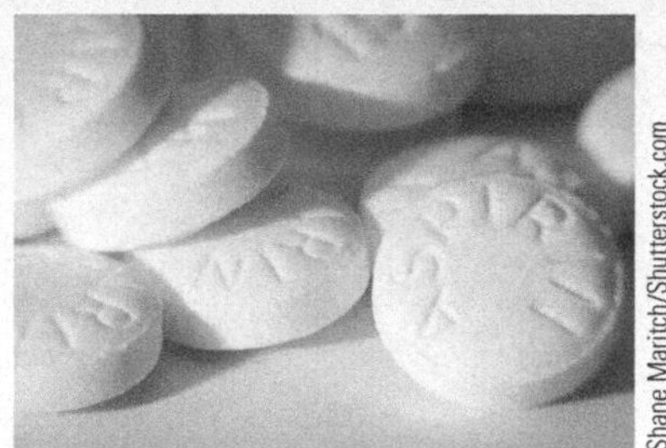 Shane Maritch/Shutterstock.com
sugar source (i.e., icing or glucose tablets)	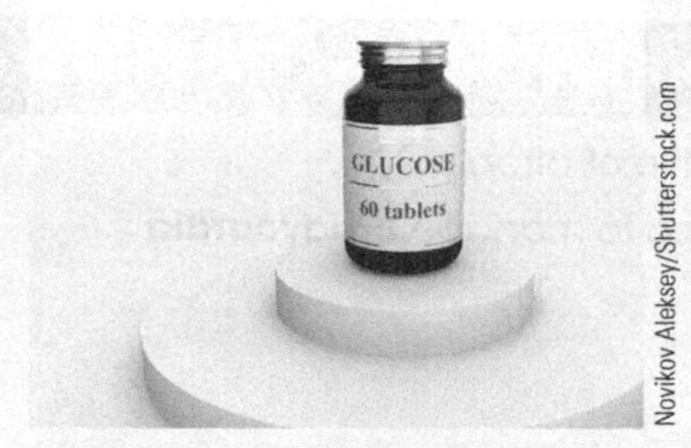 Novikov Aleksey/Shutterstock.com
histamine blocker	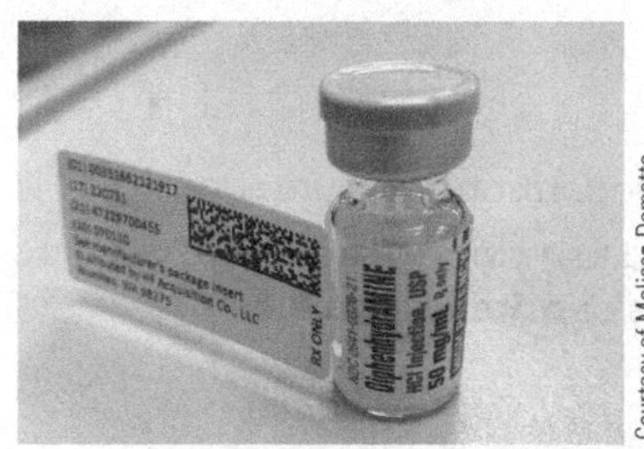 Courtesy of Melissa Damatta
12-cc disposable syringe	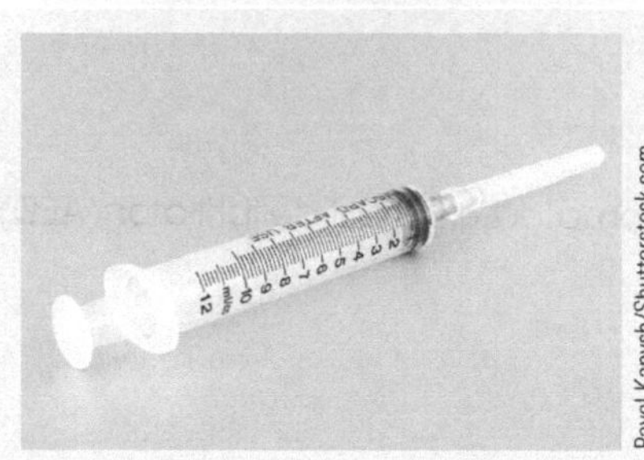 Pavel Kapysh/Shutterstock.com

(*Continued*)

TABLE 1-1 Emergency Kit Contents (*Continued*)

3-cc disposable syringe	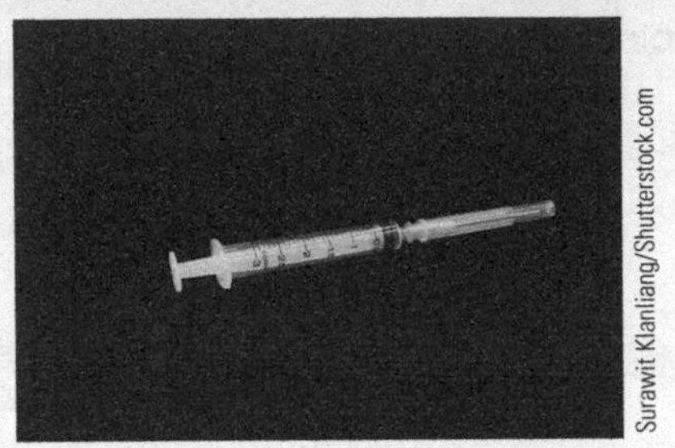 Surawit Klanliang/Shutterstock.com

TABLE 1-2 Additional Emergency Kit Contents

Bottle of atropine Used to manage **bradycardia**	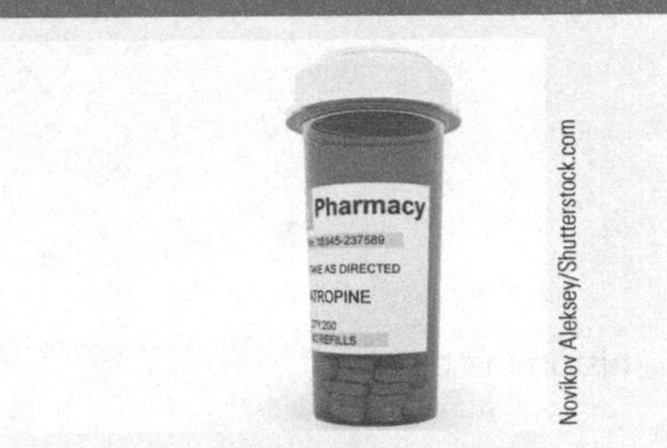 Novikov Aleksey/Shutterstock.com
hydrocortisone sodium succinate Used to manage severe allergic reactions or **adrenal insufficiency**	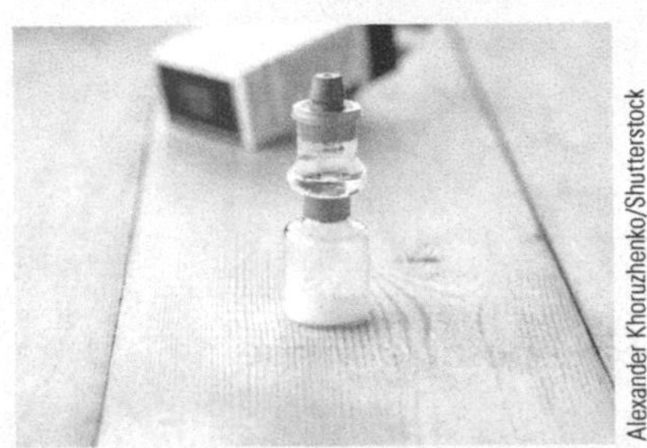 Alexander Khoruzhenko/Shutterstock
Automated external defibrillator (AED)	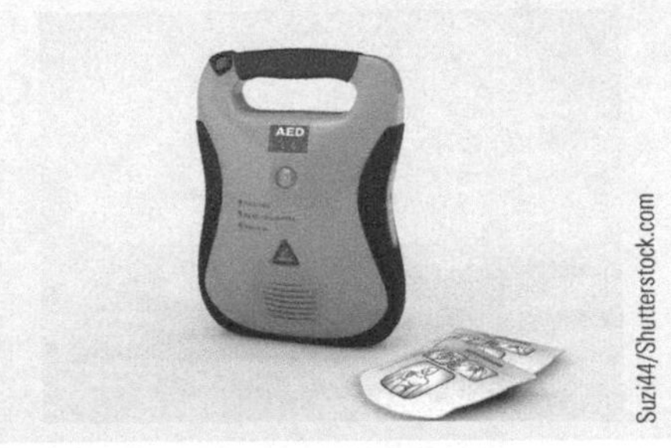 Suzi44/Shutterstock.com

TABLE 1-2 Additional Emergency Kit Contents (*Continued*)

flumazenil Used to reverse the effects of oversedation with **benzodiazepines**	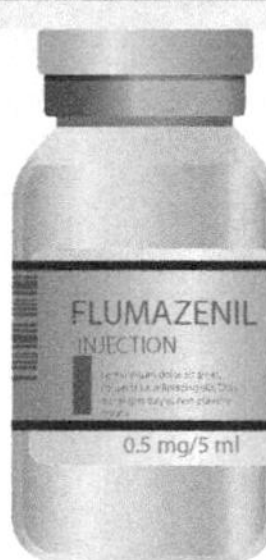
diazepam Used to treat static seizures	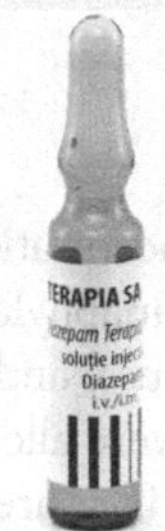 Todorean-Gabriel/Shutterstock.com
tourniquet	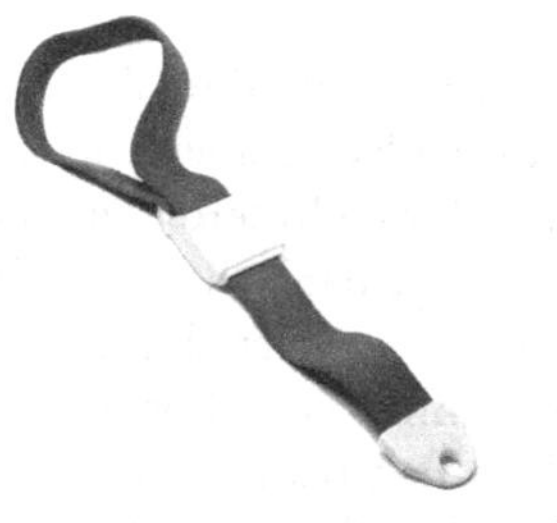 Michael Pervak/Shutterstock.com
12-gauge cricothyrotomy needle	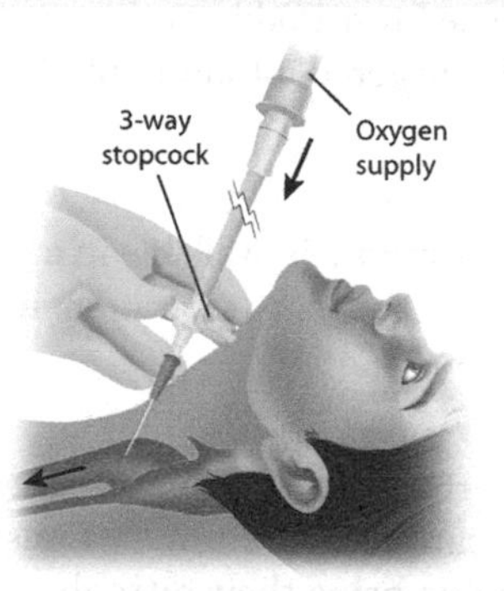

(*Continued*)

TABLE 1-2 Additional Emergency Kit Contents

airway adjuncts	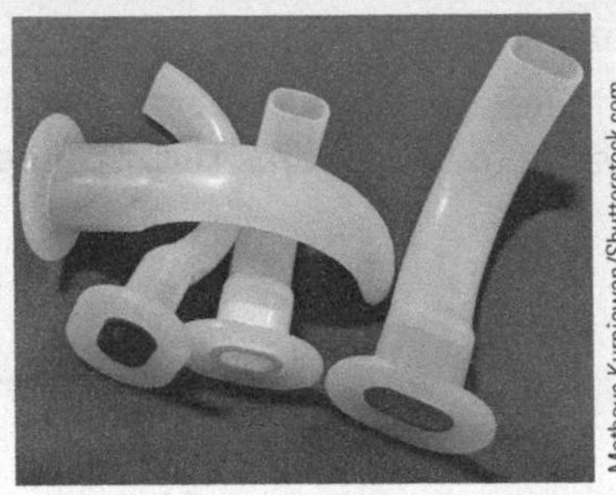 Matheus Kurniawan/Shutterstock.com

Epinephrine, injectable

Maintain a 1:1000 concentration of **epinephrine** in the emergency kit for intramuscular (IM) administration in case of an anaphylactic allergic reaction. Epinephrine is available as a preloaded syringe for rapid availability and use, and it is critical in reversing the hypotension and airway constriction that occurs during this severe allergic reaction. Epinephrine may also be used to manage an acute asthmatic reaction, which is nonresponsive to metered dose inhalers that contain a bronchodilating agent.

Bronchodilator

Bronchodilators are used to alleviate asthma symptoms and allergic reactions with symptoms of respiratory difficulty. (Epinephrine is the drug of choice for a severe anaphylactic reaction.) Bronchodilators such as **albuterol** (Proventil) relieve the constriction of asthma and allergic reactions. In asthma management, the use of bronchodilators is preferred over the use of epinephrine. The inhaler dispenses a metered dose of the bronchodilator medication upon use. Patients who have a history of asthma should bring their metered dose inhalers to their appointments. The inhaler should be kept in a readily available location in the dental operatory in the event the need arises for use. Administration should be as directed by the patient's physician. In case the administration metered dose bronchodilator does not relieve the asthma, epinephrine in a 1:1000 concentration may be administered intramuscularly.

Ammonia inhalants

Aromatic **ammonia** is available in a **vaporole** form and should be crushed and held under the patient's nose to stimulate respiration. It may be used in vasodepressor syncope.

Nitroglycerin tablets or spray

Nitroglycerine is a **vasodilator** used to manage the chest pain associated with **angina** or an acute myocardial infarction (MI) also known as heart attack. Request that patients with a history of angina bring their nitroglycerine with them. Nitroglycerine is available in a tablet form and as a sublingual spray. Tablets are the most commonly used form and have a shelf life of approximately 12 weeks once the bottle has been opened and the tablets exposed to air. The tablets are available in a .3, .4, and .6 mg dose. The sublingual spray is available as a .4 mg and .8 mg metered dose spray and has a shelf life of 2 years. Unexpired nitroglycerine, when placed under the tongue, results in a slight stinging sensation and has a bitter taste. A tablet that does not have these characteristics when placed sublingually may be expired. In such a situation in the dental office setting, the sublingual spray from the dental office emergency kit can be used to help relieve anginal pain. Three doses of nitroglycerine may be administered within a 10-minute period. If the angina pain is not relieved after nitroglycerine administration, consider the occurrence of a MI and activate EMS. Nitroglycerine's potent vasodilating activity may also be used to relieve an episode of acute hypertension. The vasodilating activity of nitroglycerine results in several transient side effects such as facial flushing, headache, and hypotension.

As part of the medical history, question male patients on the use of phosphodiesterase type 5 inhibitor (PDE5) **sildenafil** (Viagra), **tadalafil** (Cialis), and **verdanafil** (Levitra). These recently introduced medications, used to treat erectile dysfunction, are also potent vasodilators. Administration of nitroglycerine within 24 hours of ingestion of any of these PDE5 inhibitors has resulted in severe hypotensive episodes. In some cases, this drug interaction can lead to a MI and death.

Naloxone

Naloxone is the reversal agent for **opioid** sedative agents. Opioids such as codeine, oxycodone, and morphine have the ability to produce central nervous system (CNS) depression and respiratory depression. Offices administering opioids for pain management should have naloxone available for intravenous administration. The intravenous route will allow a rapid reversal of the signs and symptoms of an overdose.

Aspirin

A patient suffering from a myocardial infarction may experience signs and symptoms of pain in the chest that radiates to the left arm and shoulder, neck, and jaw. The patient may also suffer from vomiting and perspiration. Aspirin's function as an anticoagulant can aid in the management of a suspected myocardial infarction. Administration of 325 mg of aspirin in a chewable form to a conscious patient suspected of suffering from a myocardial infarction can minimize damage to the heart muscle in the area of the infarct.

Sugar source (i.e., icing)

A patient suffering from **hypoglycemia** suffers from weakness, confusion, and trembling. In case of a hypoglycemic episode, be sure to have a sugar source available in the dental office. For the conscious patient, orange juice, apple juice, non-diet soda, or chocolate may be provided to the patient. Commercial glucose tablets are also available. The signs and symptoms of hypoglycemia should rapidly reverse.

If the patient is unconscious, a liquid sugar source should not be administered. For the unconscious hypoglycemic patient, decorative cake icing should be available in the emergency kit. Cake icing may be placed in the mucobuccal fold for rapid absorption, quickly reducing the signs of hypoglycemia and producing consciousness in the patient.

Histamine blocker

An injectable **histamine** blocker such as chlorpheniramine (Chlortrimetron) or diphenhydramine (Benadryl) should be readily available in the dental emergency kit to reverse a mild to moderate **allergic** reaction. Administer these medications in liquid or dissolvable form for rapid effect. Histamine blockers do not have the ability to reverse the hypotension and airway constriction that occurs with an **anaphylactic** reaction.

It is important for the dental office to check with their state dental board for specific state requirements.

The Dental Auxiliary and the Emergency Kit

Even though it is illegal in most states for auxiliaries to use the majority of the items in the emergency kit, it is critical to be familiar with each piece of equipment and each drug in the emergency kit. The auxiliary can be of tremendous help during an emergency by promptly preparing, to the extent allowed, the correct drugs and equipment.

In addition, auxiliaries often are responsible for inspecting the emergency kit on a routine basis to check for broken equipment and expired or depleted drugs. This responsibility is assigned by the dentist as a part of the auxiliary's job description.

Drugs should always be kept updated. Administering an expired drug during an emergency can prove fatal. If the dentist wishes, arrangements can be made with certain pharmaceutical companies to replace the drugs automatically before they reach their expiration dates. If such an arrangement is made, the dates should still be double-checked by the auxiliary to prevent any errors.

The auxiliary should become familiar with the dental office's emergency kit. Kits ordered from manufacturers generally contain instructions. However, if the kit was assembled by the dentist, the auxiliary may need to obtain special instructions from other sources. If the emergency kit contains controlled substances, a method of recording the administration of these drugs should be included in the kit.

Most manufactured kits contain drugs in single-dose **ampules** (Figure 1-2). These ampules are designed to make it easy for the dental team to prepare an injection during an emergency situation. To open the ampule, hold the ampule with both hands and break it open at the color-coded line (Figure 1-3). Be careful to hold the ampule upright when breaking it open to prevent spillage. Once the ampule is open, discard the top portion and load the syringe from the remaining portion of the ampule. Some emergency drugs, for example, the EpiPen®, come preloaded. The emergency kit should always be kept in one location that is known by everyone in the office, and it should be easily accessible to everyone in the office.

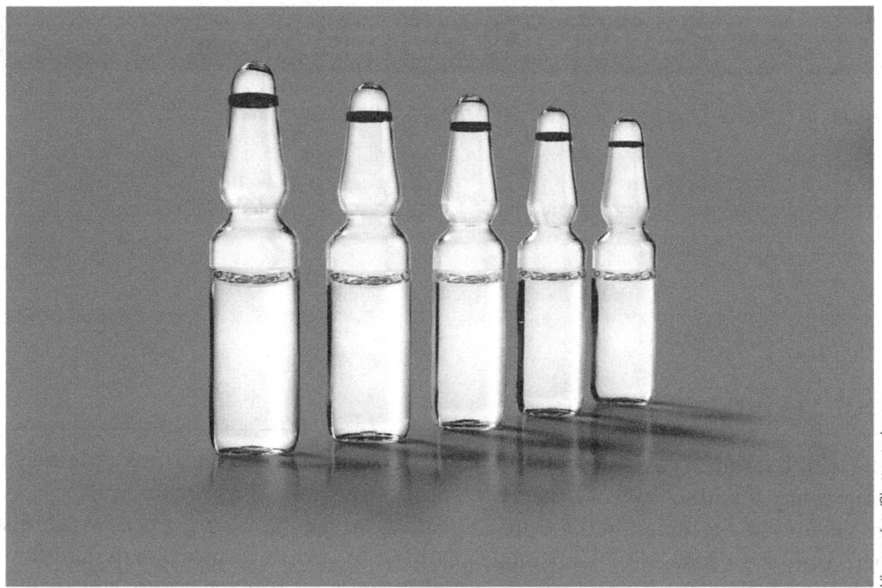

Vincenzofoto/Shutterstock.com

FIGURE 1-2 Ampules

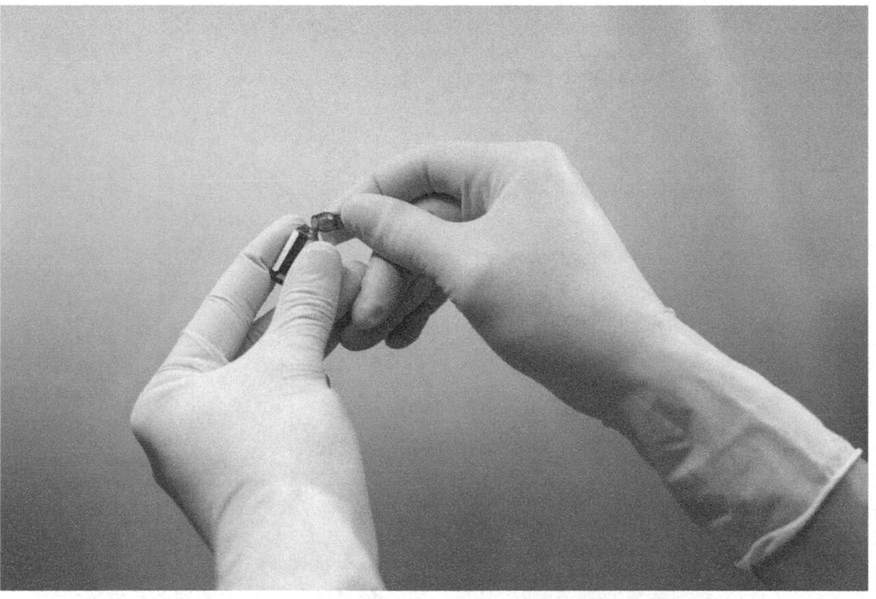

Aleksashka/Shutterstock.com

FIGURE 1-3 Breaking open ampule

TEST YOUR KNOWLEDGE

1. What is an advantage of a homemade emergency kit?

2. Where should the emergency kit be located in a dental office?

OXYGEN TANK

Oxygen is one item that can be easily administered by anyone trained in its use. It is extremely useful in most emergency situations except hyperventilation.

The oxygen comes in a cylinder. In the United States, all **oxygen tanks** are green, which distinguishes oxygen from other gases. Cylinders range in size from very large to so small that they can be carried in the hand (see Figure 1-4). Letters of the alphabet have been chosen to specify certain

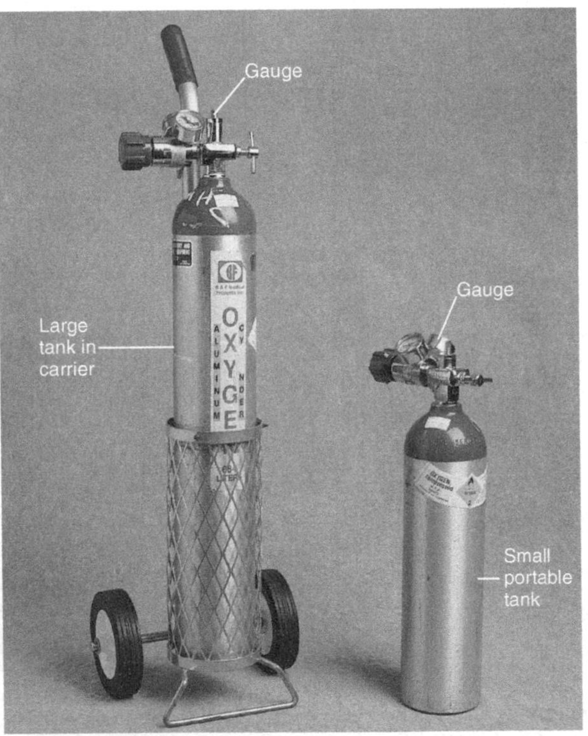

FIGURE 1-4 Oxygen tanks in varying sizes

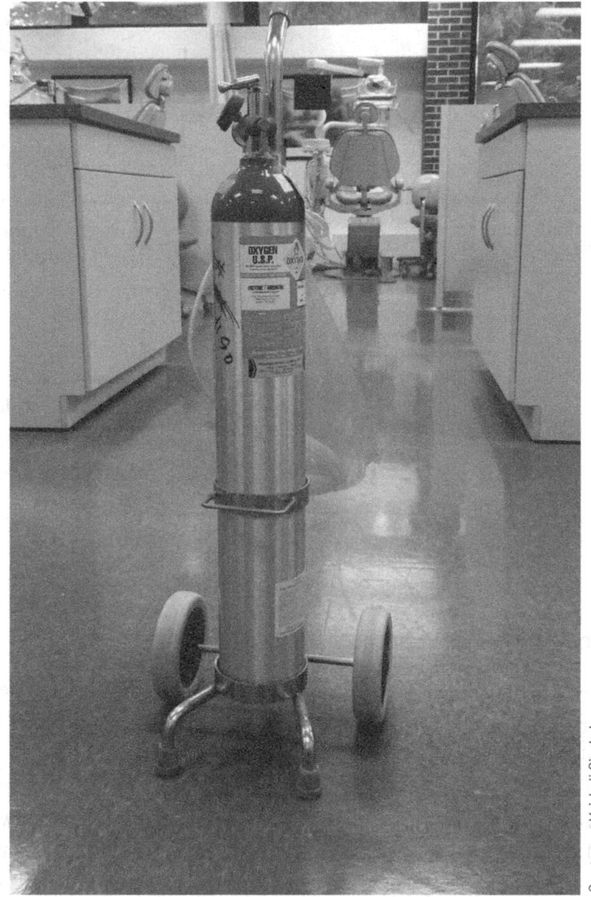

Courtesy of Vaishali Singhal

FIGURE 1-5 E-size oxygen tank

sizes of oxygen tanks; the best size for the dental office is the E cylinder (Figure 1-5). This cylinder is portable, contains about 650 liters of oxygen, and provides 100 percent oxygen for 30 minutes of constant use.

Attachments

When the oxygen tank comes from the manufacturer, it consists of only the cylinder (Figure 1-6a). A device known as a **regulator** must be attached to the tank so oxygen can be administered to the patient. The regulator is placed onto the tank to allow the pressure to be released at a reduced rate (Figure 1-6a).

Once the regulator is in place, the flow of oxygen can be adjusted by using a **flowmeter** that controls the amount of oxygen given to the patient. Two main types of flowmeters are used: the bourdon gauge flowmeter and the pressure-compensated flowmeter. The bourdon gauge consists of a round dial that indicates the flow of oxygen in liters per minute. Although it is a pressure gauge and therefore may sometimes give inadequate readings when low amounts of oxygen are being administered, it is

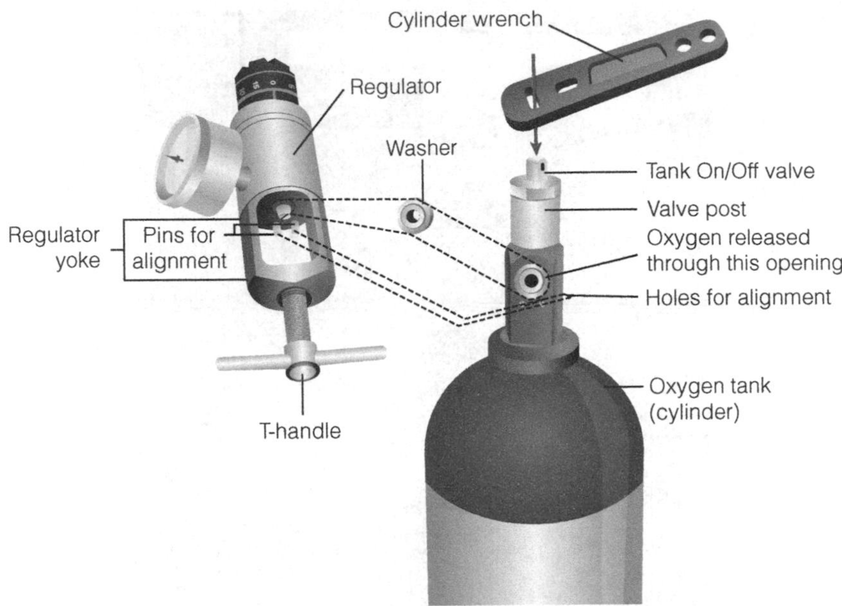

FIGURE 1-6a Oxygen tank with no regulator attached and regulator

found on a majority of tanks used in dental offices and can be functional. The pressure-compensated flowmeter consists of a vertical glass tube with a ball float that rises and falls with the flow of oxygen going through the tube (Figure 1-6b). This gauge indicates the actual flow at all times. Because it depends on the force of gravity, it must always be operated in an upright position.

While the valves and gauges on the regulator and flowmeter are necessary to release oxygen from the tank, extra attachments also are required to administer oxygen to the patient. A vast number of such attachments are available, ranging from **nasal cannulas** (see Figure 1-7) to full oxygen tents. A nasal cannula is used to deliver supplemental oxygen to a patient who needs respiratory help.

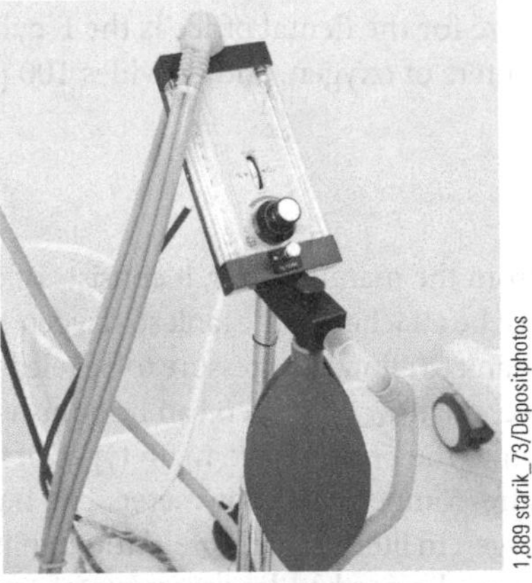
1,889 starik_73/Depositphotos

FIGURE 1-6b Flowmeter

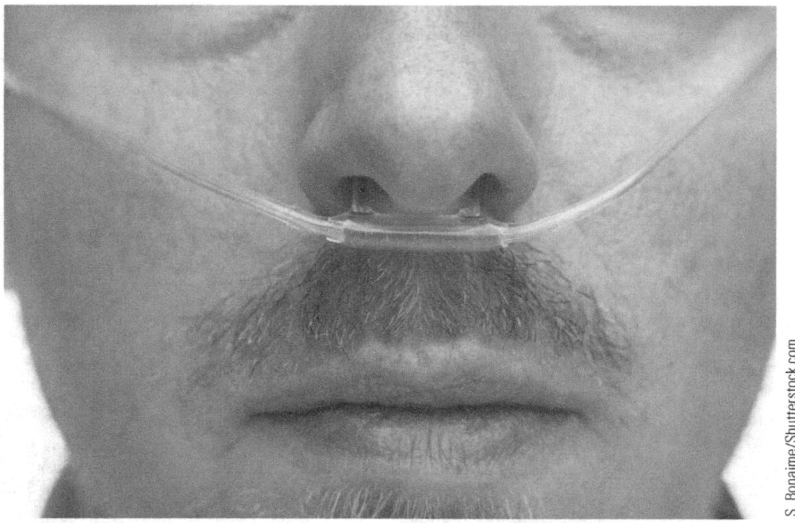

FIGURE 1-7 Nasal cannula

However, a basic **oxygen mask** (Figure 1-8) should be sufficient for administering oxygen during an emergency situation in a dental office. These attachments that allow for oxygen administration should be included in the emergency kit.

Oxygen masks are connected to the oxygen tank and are placed over the nose and mouth. They come in a variety of types and sizes designed for both adult and pediatric patients and should be available in every dental office. The mask must meet specific criteria to be effective. First, it must be the proper size and shape for the patient's face so as to provide a snug fit. Second, the mask should be made of a clear substance. It is imperative that the patient be monitored during oxygen administration to make sure they do not vomit into the mask and then aspirate the vomitus into the lungs;

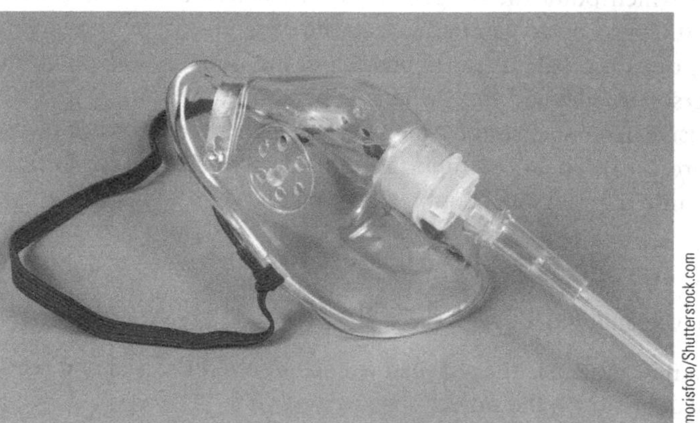

FIGURE 1-8 Clear face mask for oxygen administration; the mask should fit snugly to the patient's face for maximum effectiveness

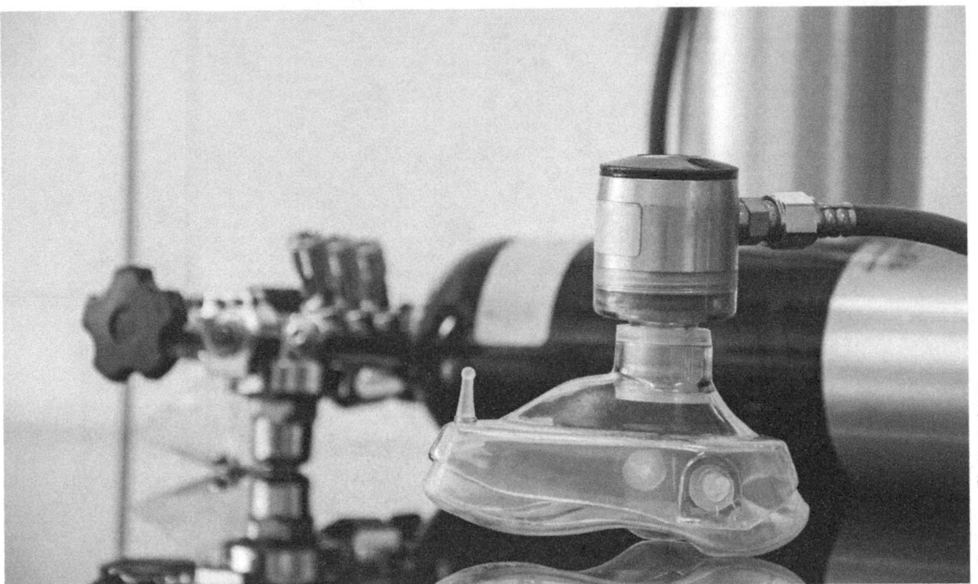

narin phapnam/Shutterstock.com

FIGURE 1-9 Oxygen tank with demand-valve resuscitation device attachment

a clear mask makes this task easier. Furthermore, with a clear mask, the person administering the oxygen can tell when the patient has started to breathe on their own because the mask will fog.

Another extremely important attachment for the office oxygen tank is the **demand-valve resuscitator** (Figure 1-9). The regular office oxygen tank is of no use to a patient who is not breathing, because there is no way to force the oxygen into the lungs. This is the function of the demand-valve resuscitator. The demand valve consists of a push button, located on the face mask, that controls the flow of oxygen. When the button is pressed, oxygen goes through the mask with enough force to inflate the lungs and is continually forced into the lungs until the valve reaches a preset pressure, at which point the oxygen stops. The demand valve is beneficial during CPR because it provides 100 percent oxygen rather than the oxygen–carbon dioxide mix a human provides. Furthermore, once the patient starts breathing, the demand valve automatically provides oxygen when the person inhales and stops when the person exhales.

Other less-expensive items such as the Ambu bag valve mask (BVM) may be used in place of the demand valve (Figure 1-10). The most important consideration is to have some mechanism available to force oxygen into the lungs of a nonbreathing patient.

Operating the Tank

When operating an oxygen tank, follow these steps:

1. When opening a new tank, use the attached wrench to open the seal and release a little oxygen to clear dust and debris from the valves.
2. Attach the regulator and flowmeter, which are designed with specific grooves and holes that can attach only one way.

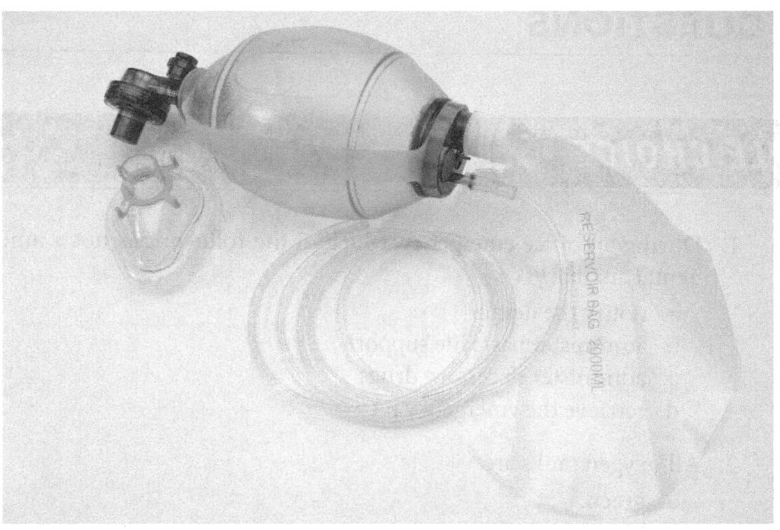

Marcin Domagala/Shutterstock.com

FIGURE 1-10 Ambu bag valve mask (BVM) resuscitation

3. Open the regulator valve all the way and then turn it back one turn. This prevents someone from thinking it is closed and damaging the equipment by turning it the wrong way.
4. Adjust the flowmeter to the point at which it is releasing 4 to 6 liters of oxygen.
5. Check the face mask hose to make sure it is not twisted or knotted.
6. Place the mask over the patient's face. Make sure the mask fits the patient with a tight seal.
7. When oxygen therapy is completed, remove the face mask, turn the flowmeter to zero, and close the tank valve. Be sure to disinfect or dispose of the mask, depending on the manufacturer's instructions.

Precautions

Although oxygen is a relatively safe gas to administer, a few precautions should be followed in the dental office:

- *Do not use oxygen near an open flame.* Oxygen is very flammable; although oxygen itself does not burn, it can cause a small flame to burn out of control.
- *Eliminate grease and oil from the area, as any kind of grease or oil can cause oxygen to combust.* Make sure you do not have oil on your hands when you operate the tank. Do not store the tank near dirty, oily rags.

SUMMARY

While not common, emergencies can occur in even the best-prepared dental office. However, a staff who knows the assigned responsibilities of each member, should have all the equipment available, should knows the emergency procedures and how to use the emergency equipment often can prevent a minor emergency from becoming a major one. The dental assistant is a vital member of the team during a medical emergency.

REVIEW QUESTIONS

MULTIPLE CHOICE

1. During an office emergency, which of the following is not a function of the dental auxiliary?
   a. notify the doctor
   b. administer basic life support
   c. administer necessary drugs
   d. retrieve the emergency kit

2. All oxygen tanks are
   a. green.
   b. blue.
   c. red.
   d. yellow.

3. The amount of oxygen the patient receives is controlled by the
   a. regulator.
   b. demand valve.
   c. cylinder.
   d. flowmeter.

4. Grease or oil should not be used around oxygen because it may
   a. contaminate the oxygen.
   b. cause combustion.
   c. block the valves.
   d. none of the above

5. Which of the following is/are true concerning the face mask on the oxygen tank?
   a. should be clear
   b. should form a tight seal
   c. should be made of metal
   d. both a and b

6. All of the following are true of the demand-valve resuscitator except one. Which is the exception?
   a. Can be used on a patient who is breathing
   b. Uses enough force to inflate the lungs
   c. Has a preset pressure
   d. Delivers 100 percent oxygen

7. A dental office may choose to have a homemade emergency kit or a manufactured emergency kit. The homemade emergency kit is usually assembled by the dentist with the help of physicians, pharmacists, and other medical personnel.
   a. Both statements are true.
   b. Both statements are false.
   c. The first statement is true, the second statement is false.
   d. The first statement is false, the second statement is true.

TRUE OR FALSE

________ 1. The emergency kit should be easily accessible to everyone in the office.

________ 2. Dental auxiliaries may administer oxygen if they are trained in its use.

________ 3. The expiration date on drugs found in the emergency kit can be checked only by the dentist.

________ 4. An E-cylinder oxygen tank should be used in the dental office.

________ 5. When administering oxygen, the flowmeter should be set on 4–6 liters.

________ 6. Since medical emergencies do not occur frequently in the dental office, it is not necessary for the dental team to carry out mock emergency drills.

MEDICAL EMERGENCY!

CASE STUDY 1-1

A 45-year-old male presents with a medical history on which he states that he has heart problems. As dental treatment begins, the patient loses consciousness and goes into cardiac arrest. The doctor sends the auxiliary to the front to call for help while the doctor goes to hook up the new oxygen cylinder that just arrived this morning. At the front desk, the assistant asks the receptionist to find the number for the emergency medical service. When the doctor and assistant return to the operatory, they begin two-person CPR with the patient in the dental chair.

Questions

1. List everything that was done incorrectly.

2. List the correct steps.

CASE STUDY 1-2

A 76-year-old female presents with a medical history on which she states that she has heart problems and diabetes. As the dental auxiliary begins to prepare the operatory, the patient loses consciousness. The dental auxiliary retrieves the emergency kit and administers several drugs to the patient. The dentist enters the operatory as the patient is regaining consciousness.

Questions

1. What did the dental auxiliary do incorrectly?

2. List the correct protocol.

CHAPTER 2

Medical History

LEARNING OUTCOMES

Upon completion of this chapter, the student will be able to:

- List the basic components of a dental patient's medical history
- Explain the rules and regulations of HIPAA
- Explain the importance of having an accurate, updated medical history for each dental patient
- Explain the technique for completing and updating the health history
- Identify the ASA classification of a patient when given a medical condition
- Utilize a drug reference manual
- Compare and contrast sources for drug references that are available to the dental auxiliary

KEY TERMS

American Society of Anesthesiologists (ASA)

ASA Physical Status Classification System

assessment

demographic

Health Insurance Portability and Accountability Act (HIPAA)

medical history

protected health information (PHI)

INTRODUCTION

Most dental office emergencies can be prevented through the use of information found on thorough medical histories. Dentists have found the easiest way to treat an emergency is to prevent it from occurring. This chapter discusses ways of gathering information from a **medical history** that may help prevent an emergency. In addition, the chapter will discuss the importance of maintaining confidentiality of information obtained from the patient.

There are a great variety of patient health history forms that are commercially available and can be purchased through various dental supply companies. Many dentists design their own forms to better suit the needs of their practice. In addition to a paper form, dental office management software companies also offer digital versions of medical histories. Some of these digital formats allow the practice to revise as they see fit. Figure 2-1a shows a sample paper medical history form and Figure 2-1b shows an example of a completed digital medical history form.

MEDICAL HISTORY FORMAT

Regardless of what type of form the dental office uses, several components are essential. First, the form should include a section for **demographic** information, including such items as name, date of birth, address, telephone number, social security number, insurance information, and person to contact in case of an emergency. The patient's primary physician should also be listed in case medical consultations are required. Next, include a detailed section pertaining to past and present medical conditions, such as surgeries, injuries, systemic diseases, current medications taken, and any known allergies. Any medical alerts, such as a known allergy to a medication or latex, should be flagged to ensure it is easily brought to the attention of the auxiliary. Figure 2-2 shows an alert that can be set up in an electronic record. The alert can be set to pop up anytime the patient record is accessed.

Last, a dental history should be included to determine any current conditions, including any chief complaints. It will also note any concerns the patient may have had with dental treatment in the past. A patient who presents with dental anxiety may be more likely to have a medical emergency than a patient who does not. Some offices may include a medical history questionnaire to help identify a patient who may have anxiety related to dental care (Table 2-1).

The section on medical conditions is very important. Each condition should be listed by its common name so it will be easily understood by the patient. The format of the medical history form should be one that allows the patient to answer questions with a yes or no and has room for follow-up questions by the auxiliary. In addition, the format should be available in multiple languages to accommodate a diverse population of patients. Medical and dental histories in various languages can be found at https://www.irvinedentalcare.com/medical-dental-history-forms/.

Completing the Medical History

The dental auxiliary or receptionist should always be available to help the patient complete the medical history. Some patients prefer to complete the forms by themselves; others may not understand

Date ______________________

PATIENT NAME	**SOCIAL SECURITY NUMBER**	**HOME PHONE** ( )
Home Address	City, State, Zip	Birthdate / /
Marital Status ❑ Single ❑ Married ❑ Divorced ❑ Separated	❑ M ❑ F	Drivers License and State

Primary Insurance Company ______________________ Group ______________ Subscriber ______________

Secondary Insurance Company ______________________ Group ______________ Subscriber ______________

Responsible Party NAME	SOCIAL SECURITY NUMBER	HOME PHONE ( )
Home Address	City, State, Zip	Birthdate / /
Marital Status ❑ Single ❑ Married ❑ Divorced ❑ Separated	Relationship to Patient	Drivers License and State
Responsible Person's Employer	Occupation	Work Phone ( )
Business Address	City	State Zip
Spouse's Name	Social Security Number	Birthdate / /
Spouse's Employer	Spouse's Occupation	Spouse's Work Phone ( )
Spouse's Business Address	City	State Zip

How did you hear about our Office?
(check only one)

Who selected this Office? ❑ Self ❑ Spouse ❑ Parent ❑ Employer

Where did you find the Phone Number to this Office? ______________________

❑ Referred by a friend	❑ Yellow Pages	❑ Relative	❑ Insurance Plan	❑ Welcome Wagon
❑ Other ____________	❑ TV/Radio Ad	❑ Newspaper Ad	❑ Direct Mailing	❑ Sign by Building

If you were referred, whom may we thank for referring you? ______________________

CONSENT

- I will answer all health questions to the best of my knowledge ________
  Initial

After explanation by the doctor, I hereby authorize the performance of dental services upon the above named patients and whatever procedures that the judgements of the doctor may decide in order to carry out these procedures. I also authorize and request the administration of any anesthetics and x-rays as may be deemed necessary and advisable by the doctor.

Signature Date Relationship to Patient

TERMS AND CONDITIONS

This office depends upon reimbursement from the patient for the costs incurred in their case. The financial responsibility of each patient must be determined before treatment.
As a condition of treatment by this office. I understand financial arrangements must be made in advance. All emergency dental services, or any dental service performed without prior financial arrangements, must be paid for at the time the services are performed.
I understand that dental services furnished to me are charged directly to me and that I am personally responsible for payment. If I carry insurance, I understand that this office will help prepare my insurance forms to assist in making collections from insurance companies and will credit such collections to my account. However, this dental office cannot render services on the assumption that charges will be paid by a insurance company.

Assignment of Insurance: I hereby authorize releases of any information needed and also authorize my insurance company to pay directly to this Office benefits accruing to me under my policy. I understand that the fee estimate listed for this dental care can only be extended for a period of 90 days form the date of the patient's examination. I also understand that in order to collect my debt, my credit history may be checked through the use of my Social Security Number or any other information I have given you. I agree that in the event that either this office or I institute any legal proceedings with respect to amount owed by me for services rendered, the prevailing party in such proceedings shall be entitled to recover all costs incurred including reasonable attorney's fees.
I grant my permission to you, or your assignee, to telephone me at home or at my work to discuss matters related to this form. I have read the above conditions and agree to their content.

Signed ______________________________ **Date** ______________

There may be a charge for any missed appointments or appointments not cancelled 48 hours before the appointment time.

FIGURE 2-1a A sample paper medical history form

PATIENTS DENTAL HEALTH

Why have you come in to see us today? (e.g.: pain, checkup, etc.) ______

Previous Dentist ______ Last Visit ______ Date of last cleaning ______

Reasons for changing dentists: ______

What problems have you had with past dental treatment? ______

Are you nervous about seeing a dentist? ☐ Yes! ☐ No If yes, please tell us why: ______

How often do you brush? ______ Do you floss? ☐ Yes ☐ No How often? ______

(please circle each)

Y N I clench or grind my teeth during the day or while sleeping.
Y N My gums bleed while brushing or flossing.
Y N I like my smile.
Y N I prefer tooth-colored fillings.
Y N I avoid brushing part of my mouth due to pain.
Y N My gums feel tender or swollen
Y N I have problems eating.
Y N I have had orthodontics.
Y N I have had a facial or jaw injury.
Y N I want my teeth straight.
Y N I want my teeth whiter.

What are your dental priorities? ______
(e.g.: apprentice, dental health, financial considerations, etc.)

PATIENTS MEDICAL HISTORY

I consider my health to be *(please check one)* ☐ Excellent ☐ Good ☐ Fair ☐ Poor

Do you or have you had any of the following? *please circle Y for yes or N for no.*

Doctor Notes Only:

1. Y N Heart Disease
2. Y N Heart Murmur/Mitral Valve Prolapse
3. Y N Stroke
4. Y N Congenital Heart Lesions
5. Y N Rheumatic Fever
6. Y N Abnormal Blood Pressure
7. Y N Anemia
8. Y N Prolonged Bleeding Disorder
9. Y N Tuberculosis or Lung Disease
10. Y N Asthma
11. Y N Hay Fever
12. Y N Sinus Trouble
13. Y N Epilepsy/Seizures
14. Y N Ulcers
15. Y N Implants/Artificial Joints: ☐ Hip ☐ Knee ☐ Other
16. Y N I smoke or use tobacco. If yes, how much per day? ______ How many years? ______
17. Y N I have consumed alcohol within the last 24 hours.
18. Y N I usually take an antibiotic prior to dental treatment.
19. Y N Have you ever taken Fen-Phen or Redux?
20. Y N I have had major surgery: Year ______ Type of operation: ______ Year ______ Type of opeartion: ______
21. Y N Do you have any other medical problem or medical history NOT listed on this form? ______
22. Y N Liver Disease
23. Y N Jaundice
24. Y N Hepatitis Type ______
25. Y N Diabetes
26. Y N Excessive Urination and/or Thirst
27. Y N Infectious Mononucleosis (Mono)
28. Y N Herpes
29. Y N Arthritis
30. Y N Sexually Transmitted/Venereal Disease
31. Y N Kidney Disease
32. Y N Tumor or Malignancy
33. Y N Cancer/Chemotherapy
34. Y N Radiation Treatment
35. Y N History of Drug Addiction
36. Y N AIDS
37. Y N Immune Suppressed Disorder
38. Y N Hearing Loss
39. Y N Fainting Spells
40. Y N Glaucoma
41. Y N History of Emotional or Nervous Disorders

WOMEN

42. Y N Are you taking birth control medication?
43. Y N Are you or could you be pregnant or nursing?

Are you allergic to any of the following?
Please circle Y for yes or N for no

44. Y N Aspirin
45. Y N Ibuprofen
46. Y N Sulfa Drugs/Sulfites/Sulfides
47. Y N Penicillin
48. Y N Codeine
49. Y N Latex, Metals, Plastics
50. Y N Local Anesthetics (Novocaine)
51. Y N Other Medications - Which ones? ______

Please list all medications you are currently taking:

Medicine ______ Condition ______
Medicine ______ Condition ______
Medicine ______ Condition ______
Medicine ______ Condition ______
Physician's Name ______ Phone ______
Address ______ Fax ______

In the event of an emergency please contact:

Name ______ Relationship ______ Phone ______
Name ______ Relationship ______ Phone ______

Initial medical/dental health reviewed by:

X ______ (Doctor's Signature) __/__/__ (Date) X ______ (Patient's Signature) __/__/__ (Date)

Periodic medical/dental health reviewed by:

X ______ (Doctor's Signature) __/__/__ (Date) X ______ (If patient is a minor: Parent/Guardian's Signature) __/__/__ (Date)

FIGURE 2-1a *(Continued)*

some of the terminology and may require assistance. Once the patient is seated in the operatory, the medical history form may be reviewed with the patient. The dental auxiliary should verbally question the patient about any positive responses as well as any conflicting answers or any unanswered questions. Positive responses are those that indicate there is a medical history problem. If there are any positive answers, the dental auxiliary will make a note next to the response on the

Time 2:39 PM | PTC_Associates | Date 3/23/2017

Eaglesoft Medical History

Patient Name: (2) Charles Abbott (Chip) Birth Date: 1/15/1978 Date Created: 8/14/2012

Although dental personnel primarily treat the area in and around your mouth, your mouth is a part of your entire body. Health problems that you may have, or medication that you may be taking, could have an important interrelationship with the dentistry you will receive. Thank you for answering the following questions.

Are you under a physician's care now?	○ Yes ◉ No	If yes
Have you ever been hospitalized or had a major operation?	○ Yes ◉ No	If yes
Have you ever had a serious head or neck injury?	○ Yes ◉ No	If yes
Are you taking any medications, pills, or drugs?	○ Yes ◉ No	If yes
Do you take, or have you taken, Phen-Fen or Redux?	○ Yes ◉ No	If yes
Have you ever taken Fosamax, Boniva, Actonel or any other medications containing bisphosphonates?	○ Yes ◉ No	If yes
Are you on a special diet?	○ Yes ◉ No	
Do you use tobacco?	○ Yes ◉ No	
Do you use controlled substances?	○ Yes ◉ No	If yes

Women: Are you...

☐ Pregnant/Trying to get pregnant? ☐ Nursing? ☐ Taking oral contraceptives?

Are you allergic to any of the following?

☐ Aspirin ☑ Penicillin ☑ Codeine ☐ Acrylic
☐ Metal ☐ Latex ☐ Sulfa Drugs ☐ Local Anesthetics

Other? ☐ If yes

Do you have, or have you had, any of the following?

AIDS/HIV Positive	○ Yes ◉ No	Cortisone Medicine	○ Yes ◉ No	Hemophilia	○ Yes ◉ No	Radiation Treatments	○ Yes ◉ No
Alzheimer's Disease	○ Yes ◉ No	Diabetes	○ Yes ◉ No	Hepatitis A	○ Yes ◉ No	Recent Weight Loss	○ Yes ◉ No
Anaphylaxis	○ Yes ◉ No	Drug Addiction	○ Yes ◉ No	Hepatitis B or C	○ Yes ◉ No	Renal Dialysis	○ Yes ◉ No
Anemia	○ Yes ◉ No	Easily Winded	◉ Yes ○ No	Herpes	○ Yes ◉ No	Rheumatic Fever	○ Yes ◉ No
Angina	○ Yes ◉ No	Emphysema	○ Yes ◉ No	High Blood Pressure	○ Yes ◉ No	Rheumatism	○ Yes ◉ No
Arthritis/Gout	○ Yes ◉ No	Epilepsy or Seizures	○ Yes ◉ No	High Cholesterol	○ Yes ○ No	Scarlet Fever	○ Yes ◉ No
Artificial Heart Valve	○ Yes ◉ No	Excessive Bleeding	○ Yes ◉ No	Hives or Rash	○ Yes ◉ No	Shingles	○ Yes ◉ No
Artificial Joint	○ Yes ◉ No	Excessive Thirst	○ Yes ◉ No	Hypoglycemia	○ Yes ◉ No	Sickle Cell Disease	○ Yes ◉ No
Asthma	◉ Yes ○ No	Fainting Spells/Dizziness	○ Yes ◉ No	Irregular Heartbeat	○ Yes ◉ No	Sinus Trouble	○ Yes ◉ No
Blood Disease	○ Yes ◉ No	Frequent Cough	○ Yes ◉ No	Kidney Problems	○ Yes ◉ No	Spina Bifida	○ Yes ◉ No
Blood Transfusion	○ Yes ◉ No	Frequent Diarrhea	○ Yes ◉ No	Leukemia	○ Yes ◉ No	Stomach/Intestinal Disease	○ Yes ◉ No
Breathing Problems	○ Yes ◉ No	Frequent Headaches	○ Yes ◉ No	Liver Disease	○ Yes ◉ No	Stroke	○ Yes ◉ No
Bruise Easily	○ Yes ◉ No	Genital Herpes	○ Yes ◉ No	Low Blood Pressure	○ Yes ◉ No	Swelling of Limbs	○ Yes ◉ No
Cancer	○ Yes ◉ No	Glaucoma	○ Yes ◉ No	Lung Disease	○ Yes ◉ No	Thyroid Disease	○ Yes ◉ No
Chemotherapy	○ Yes ◉ No	Hay Fever	◉ Yes ○ No	Mitral Valve Prolapse	○ Yes ◉ No	Tonsillitis	○ Yes ◉ No
Chest Pains	○ Yes ◉ No	Heart Attack/Failure	○ Yes ◉ No	Osteoporosis	○ Yes ○ No	Tuberculosis	○ Yes ◉ No
Cold Sores/Fever Blisters	○ Yes ◉ No	Heart Murmur	○ Yes ◉ No	Pain in Jaw Joints	○ Yes ◉ No	Tumors or Growths	○ Yes ◉ No
Congenital Heart Disorder	○ Yes ◉ No	Heart Pacemaker	○ Yes ◉ No	Parathyroid Disease	○ Yes ◉ No	Ulcers	○ Yes ◉ No
Convulsions	○ Yes ◉ No	Heart Trouble/Disease	○ Yes ◉ No	Psychiatric Care	○ Yes ◉ No	Venereal Disease	○ Yes ◉ No
						Yellow Jaundice	○ Yes ◉ No

Have you ever had any serious illness not listed above? ○ Yes ○ No If yes

Comments:

To the best of my knowledge, the questions on this form have been accurately answered. I understand that providing incorrect information can be dangerous to my (or patient's) health. It is my responsibility to inform the dental office of any changes in medical status.

Signature of Patient, Parent or Guardian:

X Charles Abbott

Date: 8/14/2012

Patterson Dental

FIGURE 2-1b A sample electronic medical history form. Note any positive answers are highlighted in red for easy identification, with response boxes to enter additional information through patient dialogue.

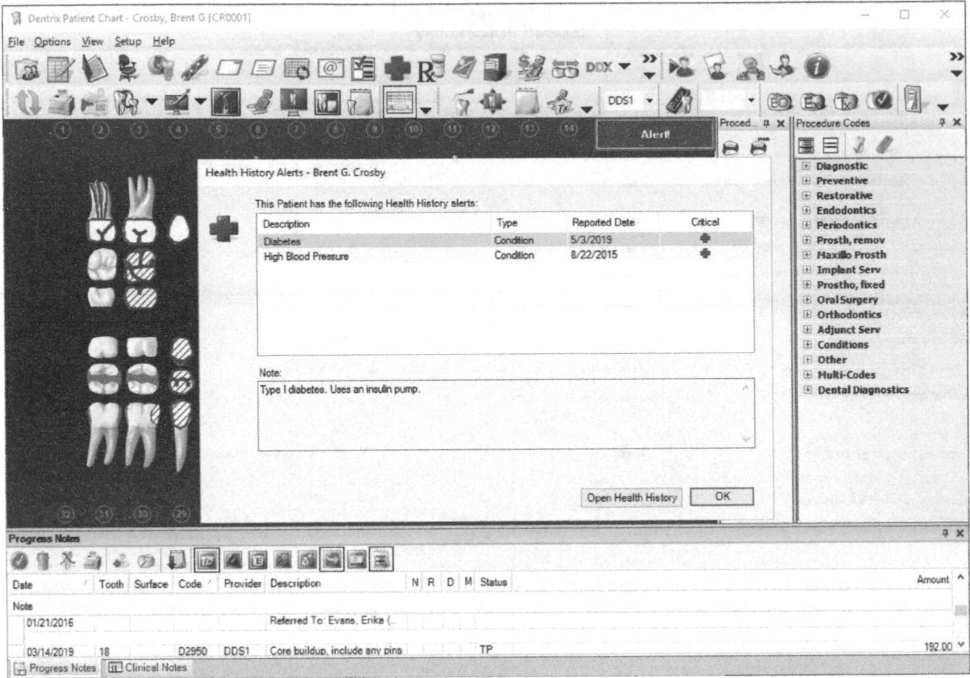

FIGURE 2-2 Electronic record alert
Source: Dentrix Dental Systems, Inc.

form if any additional information is needed. For example, if a patient gives a positive response to a history of heart disease, the dental auxiliary will ask the patient the history of the disease, if they is taking any medications and if they are under care of a cardiologist. Detailed notes should be recorded in the patient's history. Sometimes a patient will share more information regarding they medical history through conversation rather than on the medical history form. Another concern is when a patient circles an entire column of no responses. It is possible the patient did not read each selection fully. In this case, the dental auxiliary should ask the patient each question and re-circle the response, noting that it was verbally reviewed and initialed by both the dental auxiliary and patient. Figure 2-3a shows a medical history form that is improperly filled out by the patient, while Figure 2-3b shows a properly filled out medical history form.

When reviewing current medications, it is important to gather all medications including prescription, over-the-counter, and supplements/herbs. If the patient is unsure of a medication they are taking, they can bring in the prescription bottles so the proper information needed can be recorded in the patient record. Since medications can be taken for more than one condition, it may be necessary to ask the patient for what condition they are taking the medication and record it on the medical history form.

Any medical conditions that the patient reports on the medical history should be reported to the treating dentist. Furthermore, the dental auxiliary should note any medical conditions that may result in a potential medical emergency. The dental auxiliary should maintain a professional and caring manner when questioning a dental patient about current and past medical circumstances.

TABLE 2-1 Sample questionnaire to identify a patient with dental anxiety

1. How do you feel about an upcoming dental appointment?
    a. I enjoy the appointment.
    b. I am neutral about the appointment.
    c. I am somewhat anxious about the appointment.
    d. I am afraid of going to the dental office.
    e. I am extremely fearful of going to the dental office.
2. How do you feel when you are in the waiting room of the dental office?
    a. calm and relaxed
    b. slightly anxious
    c. very anxious
    d. frightened
3. How do you feel when you are in the dental chair?
    a. calm and relaxed
    b. slightly anxious
    c. very anxious
    d. frightened
4. How do you feel about the sound of the drill and other instruments?
    a. calm and relaxed
    b. slightly anxious
    c. very anxious
    d. frightened

TEST YOUR KNOWLEDGE

1. What components should be present in the medical history?
2. If a patient circles an entire column of no responses, what should the dental auxiliary do?

PATIENTS MEDICAL HISTORY

I consider my health to be *(please check one)* ☑ Excellent ☐ Good ☐ Fair ☐ Poor

Do you or have you had any of the following? *please circle Y for yes or N for no.*

1. Y N Heart Disease
2. Y N Heart Murmur/Mitral Valve Prolapse
3. Y N Stroke
4. Y N Congenital Heart Lesions
5. Y N Rheumatic Fever
6. Y N Abnormal Blood Pressure
7. Y N Anemia
8. Y N Prolonged Bleeding Disorder
9. Y N Tuberculosis or Lung Disease
10. Y N Asthma
11. Y N Hay Fever
12. Y N Sinus Trouble
13. Y N Epilepsy/Seizures
14. Y N Ulcers
15. Y N Implants/Artificial Joints: ☐ Hip ☐ Knee ☐ Other
16. Y N I smoke or use tobacco. If yes, how much per day?______ How many years?______
17. Y N I have consumed alcohol within the last 24 hours
18. Y N I usually take an antibiotic prior to dental treatment
19. Y N Have you ever taken Fen-Phen or Redux?
20. Y N I have had major surgery: Year______ Type of operation:______ Year______ Type of opeartion:______
21. Y N Do you have any other medical problem or medical history NOT listed on this form?
22. Y N Liver Disease
23. Y N Jaundice
24. Y N Hepatitis Type______
25. Y N Diabetes
26. Y N Excessive Urination and/or Thirst
27. Y N Infectious Mononucleosis (Mono)
28. Y N Herpes
29. Y N Arthritis
30. Y N Sexually Transmitted/Venereal Disease
31. Y N Kidney Disease
32. Y N Tumor or Malignancy
33. Y N Cancer/Chemotherapy
34. Y N Radiation Treatment
35. Y N History of Drug Addiction

Doctor Notes Only:

36. Y N AIDS
37. Y N Immune Suppressed Disorder
38. Y N Hearing Loss
39. Y N Fainting Spells
40. Y N Glaucoma
41. Y N History of Emotional or Nervous Disorders

WOMEN

42. Y N Are you taking birth control medication?
43. Y N Are you or could you be pregnant or nursing?

(A)

PATIENTS MEDICAL HISTORY

I consider my health to be *(please check one)* ☑ Excellent ☐ Good ☐ Fair ☐ Poor

Do you or have you had any of the following? *please circle Y for yes or N for no.*

1. Y N Heart Disease
2. Y N Heart Murmur/Mitral Valve Prolapse
3. Y N Stroke
4. Y N Congenital Heart Lesions
5. Y N Rheumatic Fever
6. Y N Abnormal Blood Pressure
7. Y N Anemia
8. Y N Prolonged Bleeding Disorder
9. Y N Tuberculosis or Lung Disease
10. Y N Asthma
11. Y N Hay Fever
12. Y N Sinus Trouble
13. Y N Epilepsy/Seizures
14. Y N Ulcers
15. Y N Implants/Artificial Joints: ☐ Hip ☐ Knee ☐ Other
16. Y N I smoke or use tobacco. If yes, how much per day?______ How many years?______
17. Y N I have consumed alcohol within the last 24 hours
18. Y N I usually take an antibiotic prior to dental treatment
19. Y N Have you ever taken Fen-Phen or Redux?
20. Y N I have had major surgery: Year______ Type of operation:______ Year______ Type of opeartion:______
21. Y N Do you have any other medical problem or medical history NOT listed on this form?
22. Y N Liver Disease
23. Y N Jaundice
24. Y N Hepatitis Type______
25. Y N Diabetes
26. Y N Excessive Urination and/or Thirst
27. Y N Infectious Mononucleosis (Mono)
28. Y N Herpes
29. Y N Arthritis
30. Y N Sexually Transmitted/Venereal Disease
31. Y N Kidney Disease
32. Y N Tumor or Malignancy
33. Y N Cancer/Chemotherapy
34. Y N Radiation Treatment
35. Y N History of Drug Addiction

Doctor Notes Only:

36. Y N AIDS
37. Y N Immune Suppressed Disorder
38. Y N Hearing Loss
39. Y N Fainting Spells
40. Y N Glaucoma
41. Y N History of Emotional or Nervous Disorders

WOMEN

42. Y N Are you taking birth control medication?
43. Y N Are you or could you be pregnant or nursing?

(B)

FIGURE 2-3 Medical histories filled out by the patient. (a) Medical history improperly filled out and (b) Medical history properly filled out

Confidentiality of the Medical History

As with any other information obtained in the dental office, the information on medical history is confidential. The information obtained on the medical history should be made available only to authorized users with the patient's full consent. In 1996, the **Health Insurance Portability and Accountability Act (HIPAA)** was signed into federal law. The rules and regulations of HIPAA define how sensitive information obtained from the patient can be circulated and to whom the information can be distributed with the patient's written consent and knowledge. A portion of HIPAA, known as the privacy rules, establishes rules and regulations for the protection of **protected health information** (PHI). Today, more providers are moving toward electronic dental records. To allow practices to adopt these new technologies while still ensuring the safety of the transmission of these records, the security rule was developed. The security rule sets standards on how to protect patient private health information that is transferred through electronic forms.

Updating the Health History

The health history should be updated at each visit to the office. A person's medications and medical condition can change between visits, and it is extremely important to keep this information current. The dental auxiliary will verbally update the health history with the patient and document the patient's response with the date in the patient's record.

TEST YOUR KNOWLEDGE

1. When should a medical history be updated?
2. What is PHI?

ASSESSMENT OF THE DENTAL PATIENT

To prevent an emergency from occurring, it is important for the dental auxiliary to take into account the dental patient's general health status. An **assessment** of the dental patient consists of reviewing the medical history and the likely side effects of any prescribed medications. After this information is evaluated, the patient can be placed into a physical classification based on the **American Society of Anesthesiologists** (ASA) classification system shown in Table 2-2. This helps the dentist evaluate possible risks and outcomes pertaining to the treatment to be provided. When evaluating a patient's risk, the dental team is usually dealing with only the first four ASA classifications in the **ASA Physical Status Classification System**. However, if the patient is a Class IV ASA status, any elective procedures should be postponed until the patient can be classified as a Class III. If an emergency presents, a Class IV may be treated conservatively and in the most noninvasive way. Management is based on the type of emergency taking place. Each emergency and its management will be discussed in subsequent chapters of this text.

TABLE 2-2 ASA Physical Status Classifications

ASA Class	Description	Examples (including but not limited to)
I	Healthy patient	None
II	Patient with well-controlled mild systemic disease	Well-controlled diabetes and well-controlled hypertension, mild stable angina
III	Patient with severe systemic disease	Poorly controlled diabetes and hypertension, COPD, morbidly obese (BMI >40), on regular dialysis, history of myocardial infarction or cerebrovascular accident (>3 months), stable angina
IV	Patient with severe systemic disease that is a constant threat to life	Recent myocardial infarction or cerebrovascular accident (<3 months), severe valve dysfunction, unstable angina
V	Moribund patient who is not expected to survive more than 24 hours	End stage renal disease, end stage cancer, end stage AIDS

Source: American Society of Anesthesiologists "https://www.asahq.org/~/media/sites/asahq/files/public/resources/standards-guidelines/asa-physical-status-classification-system.pdf

USING DRUG REFERENCES

The dental auxiliary should research and record any information about the medications that are prescribed by the patient's physician or other health care provider. The dental auxiliary should note what medical condition each medication is prescribed for, and specifically call attention to any side effects of the medications, especially ones that have dental implications. Reviewing the medical history is extremely valuable to the entire dental team in understanding existing medical conditions, preventing the use of medications that may be contraindicated, and determining if there are restrictions on the type of treatment that may be provided to the patient.

All information determined by reviewing the patient's medical history should be described to the dentist so that they can ultimately determine how the patient's treatment will be accomplished to minimize the potential for emergencies. As a result of obtaining the information, it is sometimes necessary to consult the patient's physician or specialist to determine possible medical risks with any dental treatment.

Several sources may be used to obtain medication information. The dentist and staff should decide which source best meets the needs of their office.

TABLE 2-3 PDR Sections

Section	Description
I	Manufacturer's index. Useful to use if the need to contact a manufacturer should arise
II	Page numbers for medications listed by generic and brand names
III	Lists therapeutic class and sub-classes, action of the drug (i.e., blood thinner)
IV	Photo identification in color
V	Detailed medication information (i.e., dosage, side effects); information commonly seen on a package insert
VI	Diagnostic product information

Using the *Physician's Desk Reference*

One drug reference source is the ***Physician's Desk Reference (PDR)***. The *PDR* is compiled annually and contains information provided by the drug manufacturers about a large variety of medications. There are six sections that are color coded and may be of value to the auxiliary. Table 2-3 lists the six sections with their descriptions included in the *PDR*. Complete instructions on how to use the *PDR* are provided at the beginning of each section. See Figure 2-4.

The product identification section provides pictures of a wide variety of medications. Often patients come to the office with pill boxes containing a variety of medications, but they do not know the names of the medications or the conditions for which the medications have been prescribed. This section of the *PDR* allows the auxiliary to visually identify the medication.

The *PDR* is not the only general medication reference book. Another great resource to use for drug identification is the *Delmar Healthcare Drug Handbook*, which is updated annually as well.

Other drug reference sources are published for specific specialties in medicine, such as dentistry. One such example is the *Dental Drug Reference with Clinical Implications*. These guides place emphasis on dental considerations during treatment as well as common oral side effect of the medications. This becomes quite valuable as it allows for a rapid response when reviewing the patient's medication history that could have implications for dental care. See Figure 2-5.

Finally, electronic versions of drug reference manuals are available through online resources, CD/DVD sources, and applications. Caution should be used to determine the accuracy as well as the completeness of the information.

Even though it is ultimately the dentist's responsibility to make all decisions regarding the patient's medications, it is important for the auxiliary to know as much as possible about the patient to assist in providing proper treatment. The auxiliary should become familiar with the contents of the drug reference source selected and should use it regularly. It is extremely important to have an up-to-date resource, because medications change at such a rapid pace.

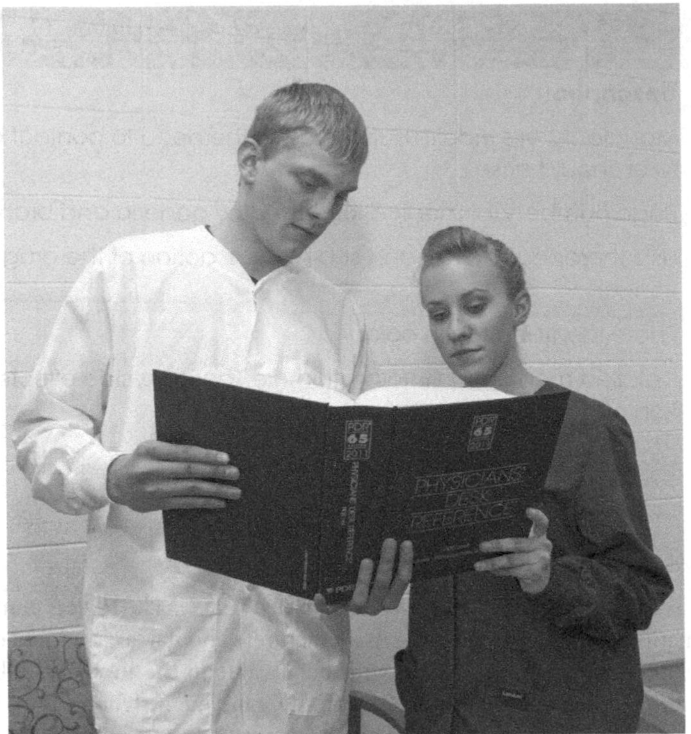

FIGURE 2-4 Dental auxiliaries reviewing the Physicians Desk Reference.

After the dental auxiliary has reviewed the medical history and the list of prescribed medications, a determination of whether the patient's medical history is positive or negative is needed. A positive medical history would be one in which the patient presents with single or multiple medical conditions along with accompanying prescribed medications. A negative medical history would be one in which the patient presents with a no history of medical conditions and no prescribed medications.

TEST YOUR KNOWLEDGE

1. What ASA classifications would not allow for elective dental treatment?

2. What are examples of electronic drug reference sources?

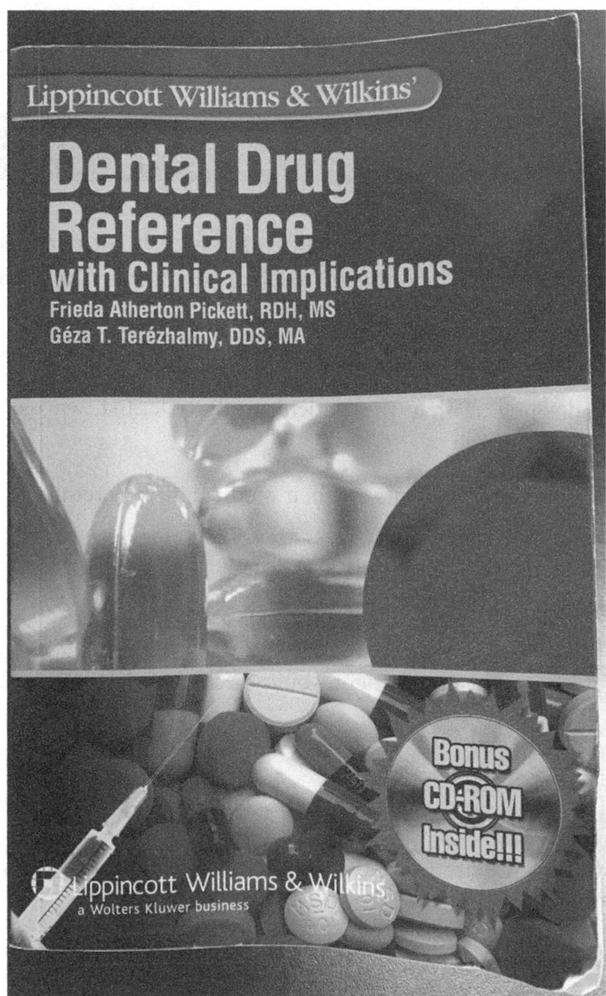

FIGURE 2-5 Dental drug reference guide
Source: Lipincott, Williams & Wilkins

SUMMARY

When a new patient enters the dental office, the staff and dentist do not know the types of medical problems the patient has. When we think of treating the patient, we want to employ the idea to never treat a stranger. If a thorough health history is not obtained and an emergency were to arise, there would be no point of reference on which to base a probable diagnosis on the emergency at hand. The medical history informs the staff about possible problems for which to prepare as well as which medications and treatments to avoid. When the dental team has all this information available, the doctor and staff have taken the first step toward preventing a serious dental office emergency.

REVIEW QUESTIONS

MULTIPLE CHOICE

1. If a dental patient has difficulty with english, the dental auxiliary should
   a. Make an appointment for the patient when the services of an interpreter are available.
   b. Have medical histories available in different languages.
   c. Speak louder so that the patient will understand.
   d. Suggest that the patient find a dentist who speaks their primary language.

2. Interviewing patients for their medical history requires
   a. special credentials.
   b. good communication skills.
   c. good computer skills.
   d. a lot of time and energy.

3. A normal healthy patient would be classified as which of the following?
   a. ASA I
   b. ASA II
   c. ASA III
   d. ASA IV

4. A patient with a severe systemic disease would be classified as which of the following?
   a. ASA I
   b. ASA II
   c. ASA III
   d. ASA IV

5. Which of the following is not a component of the patient's medical history?
   a. date of birth
   b. address
   c. phone number
   d. ethnic background

6. The rules and regulations of HIPAA define how sensitive information obtained from the patient can be circulated and to whom the information can be distributed with the patient's written consent and knowledge. A portion of

HIPAA, known as the privacy rules, establishes rules and regulations for the protection of **protected health information (PHI)**.

Select the correct response based on the statement above.

a. Both statements are true.
b. Both statements are false.
c. The first statement is true, the second statement is false.
d. The second statement is false, the first statement is true.

7. Which of the following is correct regarding the *PDR*?
   a. It Is updated every 6 months.
   b. It has four sections so medications can be looked up in different ways.
   c. The PDR is the only general medication reference book available.
   d. Drug references are available in digital format.

8. Which of the following is not correct regarding a patient's medical history?
   a. Negative responses mean that there is a medical problem or concern
   b. There is no need to discuss the medical history with the patient as long as the form Is completely filled out
   c. Any medical alerts should be flagged in the computer system
   d. The dental auxiliary does not need to be available to help the patient complete the form.

9. A patient with a well-controlled mild systemic disease is which of the following ASA Classifications?
   a. ASA I
   b. ASA II
   c. ASA III
   d. ASA IV

10. HIPAA establishes rules and regulations for the protection of personal health information. If an office uses digital records, HIPAA laws do not apply.

    Select the correct response based on the statement above.

    a. Both statements are true.
    b. Both statements are false.
    c. The first statement is true, the second statement is false.
    d. The second statement is false, the first statement is true.

TRUE OR FALSE

_______ 1. The health history should be obtained only with emergency patients.

_______ 2. The health history should be updated each time the patient comes to the office.

_______ 3. The *PDR* should be replaced every year.

_______ 4. An ASA V classification patient would be commonly seen in a dental office for dental treatment.

_______ 5. The dental history is not considered to be part of the medical history.

_______ 6. HIPAA allows the dental practitioner to share patient personal health information to anyone that requests it.

_______ 7. Drug references that are specific to dentistry are not available, so the best source is the *PDR*.

_______ 8. The patient's address should be included as part of the medical history.

_______ 9. The patient's city of birth should be inlcuded as part of the medical history.

_______ 10. According to HIPAA laws, patient health information can be distributed without written permission from the patient.

MEDICAL EMERGENCY!

CASE STUDY 2-1

A 27-year-old female presents at the dental office for an initial exam. After the dental auxiliary reviews the medical history and records the vital signs, she notifies the dentist that the patient has a history of poorly controlled diabetes.

Questions

1. What ASA classification would fit this patient?

2. Would she have a positive or negative medical history? Why?

3. Which drug reference may be useful to look up the dental implications of the patient's medications?

CASE STUDY 2-2

A 56-year-old male presents at the dental office for a restorative appointment. After reviewing the medical history and recording the vital signs, the dental auxiliary notifies the dentist that the patient has had a change in his medical history. He is no longer being treated for hypertension due to improvement through diet and exercise.

Questions

1. What ASA classification would fit this patient?
2. Would he have a positive or negative medical history? Why?

CHAPTER 3

Vital Signs

LEARNING OUTCOMES

Upon completion of this chapter, the student will be able to:

- Define key terms
- Name the four primary vital signs
- Determine when the two additional vital signs may be necessary to monitor for patient treatment
- Demonstrate the technique for obtaining each of the four primary vital signs
- Explain the normal range of each of the four primary vital signs
- Explain why determining baseline vital signs is important in assessing a patient's health status
- Record all four primary vital signs

KEY TERMS

antecubital fossa
arrhythmia
baseline vital signs
blood pressure
bradypnea
carotid artery
diastolic blood pressure
hypertension
Korotkoff sounds
nosocomial
pulse
radial artery
respiration rate
sphygmomanometer
stethoscope
systolic blood pressure
tachycardia
tachypnea

VITAL SIGNS

The human body has four vital signs that are important to measure: *blood pressure, pulse, respiration rate*, and *temperature*. Additionally, height and weight can be recorded especially if these observations are important in the patient's treatment. For example, in pediatric dentistry, height and weight for a child is necessary for the prescribing of medication.

Vital signs are clinical observations that are made to discover the patient's health condition, both physically and mentally. These clinical findings may provide the dental auxiliary and dentist with information on how the patient may respond to treatment. The vital signs vary depending on the age, gender, weight, and physical health of the patient. Since the patient is usually less apprehensive at the initial consultation visit, it is important to record vital signs at this time. Furthermore, the observation and recording of initial or **baseline vital signs** prior to any dental treatment can help the staff determine how the patient is responding during the dental procedure and can be used for reference in the event an emergency occurs. This chapter discusses ways of obtaining the four primary vital signs and the significance of these vital signs in the dental setting.

BLOOD PRESSURE

Blood pressure is the pressure the blood places on the walls of the arteries. It is recorded in units of millimeters of mercury, or "mm Hg," and expressed as two numbers, for example, 120/80. The upper number (in this case, 120) is the **systolic blood pressure**. This is the pressure required for the left ventricle to pump the blood to the remaining vessels in the body. The lower number (in the example above, 80) is the **diastolic blood pressure**. This number is the pressure of the heart muscle at rest while it is refilling with blood.

When there is too much pressure on the arteries, the patient develops **hypertension**, also known as high blood pressure. Hypertension can result in serious conditions such as stroke or cardiac arrest. By measuring blood pressure, the dentist can prevent an emergency from occurring in the dental office. It also serves as a screening tool for the patient, helping to recognize an undiagnosed condition of hypertension.

Based on American Dental Association (ADA) recommendations, blood pressure should be obtained at the initial visit for each new patient as a screening tool for undiagnosed hypertension. If an elevated blood pressure is obtained, notify the patient, wait 5–10 minutes, and take a second reading. Record both readings in the chart. At the next appointment, a third reading should be obtained. If all three readings are elevated, it is possible that the patient may be suffering from undiagnosed hypertension and should be referred to their physician for further evaluation. If the blood pressure is extremely high (Stage 2 according to Table 3-1), it may not be safe to treat the patient at that visit. Patients with uncontrolled hypertension are at a higher risk for a cardiovascular accident. Elective care should be postponed until the blood pressure has been brought under control by a physician.

To measure blood pressure, two items are needed: a **stethoscope** and a **sphygmomanometer** (see Figure 3-1). The sphygmomanometer, which consists of a gauge and an inflatable bag inside a cloth armband, is available in a range of sizes designed to fit children and adults. The cuff should always be selected according to the patient's size rather than the patient's age. It is essential that the patient be relaxed and that an appropriately sized blood pressure cuff be used. Large cuffs may be used for blood pressure measurements on larger patients and pediatric-sized cuffs are available for

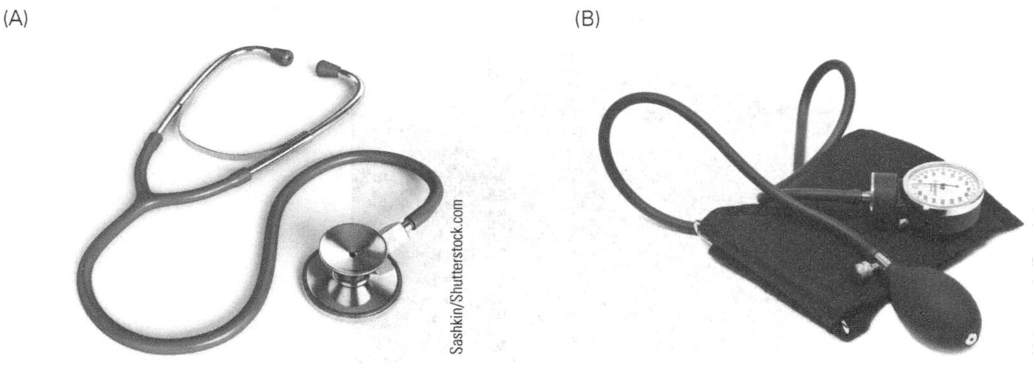

FIGURE 3-1 (a) stethoscope; (b) sphygmomanometer

use on children and small adults. An inappropriately sized cuff will produce inaccurate readings. Either the right or the left arm may be used to record the blood pressure; however, blood pressure in the right arm will usually be approximately 10 mm Hg lower than in the left arm.

TEST YOUR KNOWLEDGE

1. What four primary vital signs are recorded in a dental office?

2. The blood pressure reading is represented by two numbers. What are these numbers called?

Technique

Blood pressure is measured by comparing the pressure in the artery with the air pressure in the armband using the following steps.

- Assemble armamentarium: sphygmomanometer, stethoscope, medical history form.
- Wash and dry hands.
- Greet patient and introduce self.
- Explain procedure and purpose to patient.
- The patient should be seated with the arm at heart level and elbow supported on a surface at heart level, with legs uncrossed and back and feet supported.
- Support elbow on a solid surface.
- Remove all air from the sphygmomanometer by squeezing the cuff.

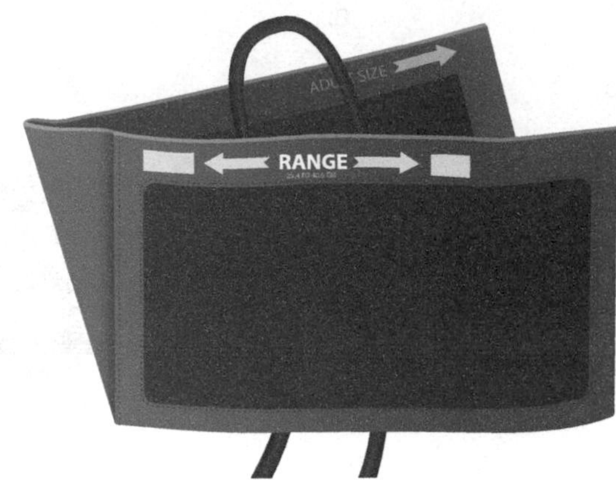

FIGURE 3-2 Range markings on cuff for accurate sizing

- Expose the patient's arm. An accurate blood pressure cannot be taken over any type of clothing.
- Select the cuff size. Be sure to select a size that fits snugly around the patient's arm without being tight enough to stop the flow of blood. A cuff that is too large or too small may produce an inaccurate reading. Some cuffs will have range markings (see Figure 3-2) to ensure an accurate fit.
- Place the cuff approximately an inch above the **antecubital fossa** (Figure 3-3), with gauge visible to operator (Figure 3-4).
- Close the small knob on the bulb by turning it clockwise. Make sure that the knob is not so tight as to prevent it from being easily turned with two fingers (Figure 3-4).

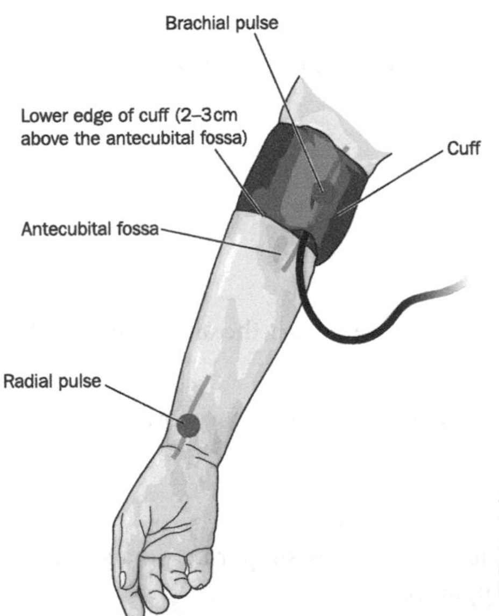

FIGURE 3-3 Location of the antecubital fossa

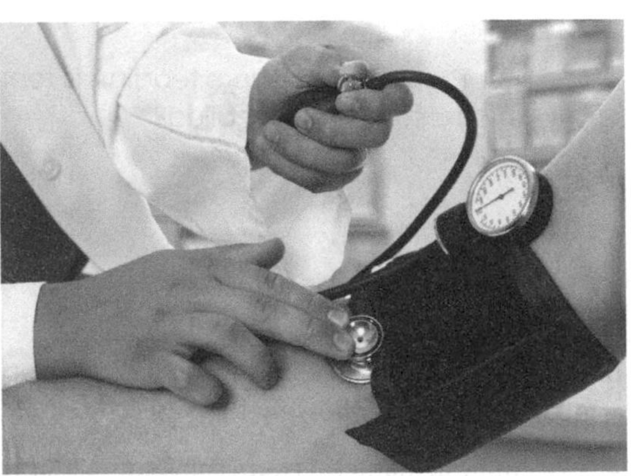

FIGURE 3-4 Turn the knob on the blood pressure cuff

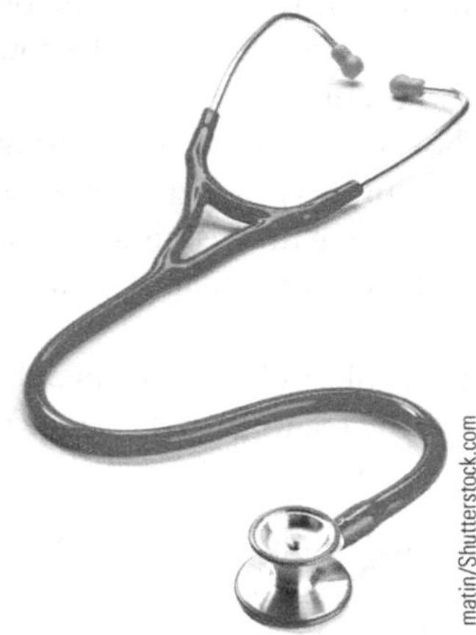

FIGURE 3-5 Placement of the ear tips pointed forward

- Place eartips of the stethoscope in your ears; be sure that they are facing toward (see Figure 3-5) the front. This will allow for a better fit and a more comfortable placement as they follow the shape of the ear canal.
- Place the bell of the stethoscope over the brachial artery in the antecubital fossa.
- Squeeze the bulb to pump air into the cuff until the pressure stops the flow of blood in the artery. This can be determined by palpating the **radial artery** (see Figure 3-6). When no pulse is felt, the flow of blood has been stopped; this is the palpatory radial systolic reading. The cuff should be inflated 20–30 mm Hg above the palpatory radial systolic reading.

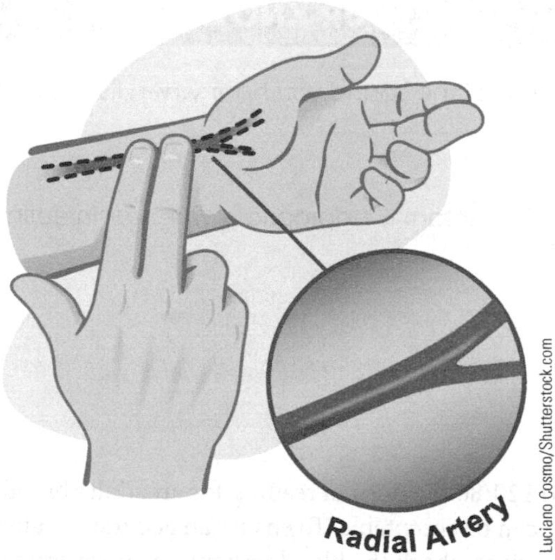

FIGURE 3-6 Measuring the pulse at the radial artery

- Turn the knob on the bulb counterclockwise slowly to release the pressure in the cuff. If the pressure is released too rapidly, you will be unable to hear the pulse sound. If this occurs, release all the pressure in the cuff and begin the procedure again.
- As soon as the cuff is loose enough to allow the blood to pass through the artery, you should begin to hear sounds known as **Korotkoff sounds**. These are various heart sounds such as thuds and swishes that are a result of the blood reentering the vessels as the pressure of the cuff is being released. They are heard in five phases. At phase 1, you will hear a thud. At this point the reading on the gauge is the systolic pressure.
- Continue to release the pressure in the cuff until a pulse is no longer heard. This is phase 5, and at this point the blood is flowing freely, and the reading on the gauge is the diastolic pressure.
- Record blood pressure on medical history form.

The technique described here is only one example of how to measure blood pressure. If you are in an office that uses a different technique, make sure you understand the steps involved and can perform the procedure accurately. Many dental offices use one of the different types of digital blood pressure cuffs that are available. When using a digital cuff, follow the manufacturer's instructions carefully to use the cuff effectively and to accurately record the reading.

Disinfection of stethoscopes

Studies have found that the majority of stethoscopes are contaminated and as a result may transmit **nosocomial** infections. Isopropyl alcohol may be used to disinfect stethoscopes regularly and is less corrosive to the metal and rubber components of this instrument than other germicides.

Beginning with the earpieces, wipe the stethoscope, including the bell and diaphragm. To thoroughly wipe the diaphragm, take it apart to remove any particles by wiping with an alcohol gauze and then reassemble.

TEST YOUR KNOWLEDGE

1. What is the name of the sound you hear when listening to blood pressure called?
2. What type of disinfectant is appropriate when disinfecting the stethoscope?

Normal Readings

Physicians once considered 120/80 the normal reading for an adult's blood pressure, but many now believe that a lower reading can be acceptable. To ensure an accurate reading and to determine what is normal for a particular patient, check the blood pressure over several visits. In addition, consult with the patient's physician if indicated. For example, if the dentist feels that the patient's health may

TABLE 3-1 Blood Pressure Categories for Dental Offices

	Systolic (mm Hg)		Diastolic (mm Hg)
Normal	Less than 120	and	Less than 80
Elevated	120–129	or	Less than 80
Hypertension Stage 1	130–139	or	80–89
Hypertension Stage 2	140 and above	or	90 and above

Source: Adapted from the American Heart Association Guidelines, 2017.

be affected in any negative manner, a physician's consultation may be necessary before any dental treatment is performed.

Clinical management of a patient with hypertension may require some modification in treatment. It is important to ensure good pain management techniques and implement stress reduction protocol. Short appointments will be less stressful for patients with hypertension. Nitrous oxide and oxygen sedation for relaxation will be beneficial. Use of epinephrine in the local anesthetic should be limited to .4 mg or 2 cartridges of lidocaine with 1:100,000 epinephrine concentration.

When recording a patient's blood pressure, note the extremity used (e.g., arm or leg). Also note whether the right or left side has been used, as well as the position of the patient. Such a reading, for example, could be written as follows: 120/80 R arm sitting. See Table 3-1 for blood pressure categories used in the dental office setting.

RECORDING THE PULSE

The **pulse** is an important measurement to obtain on each dental patient. As with any vital sign, it is important to have a baseline reading for comparison in the event of an emergency.

The pulse can be measured at any major artery in the body. The most common artery to use to record pulse in a dental office setting is the radial artery (Figure 3-3) in the wrist, as it provides easy access and an accurate reading. The **carotid artery** located on either side of the neck (Figure 3-6) may also be used and is the preferred artery during a medical emergency because it supplies the blood to the brain and the head. When cardiac output is low because of an emergency condition, the pulse may not be palpable at the radial artery (since the radial artery is peripheral, blood flow usually ceases in that area first). In this situation, measure the pulse at the carotid artery for more accuracy.

Technique

To record the pulse correctly, use the first and middle fingers in measuring it (Figure 3-7). Place the two fingers firmly over the artery. Placing the fingers too lightly will cause you to miss the

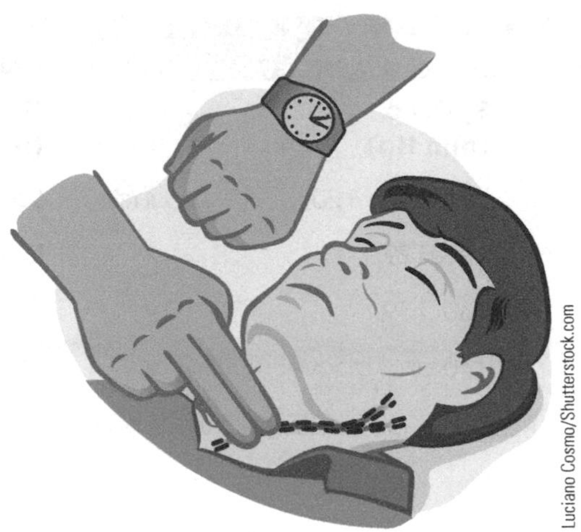

Luciano Cosmo/Shutterstock.com

FIGURE 3-7 Measuring the pulse at the carotid artery

beat of the pulse; pressing too tightly will cut off the blood supply, eliminating the pulse altogether. The thumb should not be used to for taking this recording, because the thumb has its own pulse.

Once the artery has been located, count each beat of the pulse for a full minute. Observing the second hand of a watch is mandatory. Although the rate or speed of the pulse is important, attention also must be paid to the rhythm (regular or irregular) and to the quality (bounding or thready). Each of these readings is important to the dentist in diagnosing the problem during an emergency. Although normal pulse readings vary among patients, for an adult the average range is 60 to 80 beats per minute (bpm). A pulse that is fast may be a sign of **tachycardia** (rapid heart rate); a slow pulse rate may be a sign of bradycardia (slow heart rate). A pulse with an abnormal rhythm may signify an **arrhythmia** (abnormal heart rhythm). Medications may also cause a change in the pulse rate. The cause of an abnormal pulse rate should be investigated to determine cause. Patients

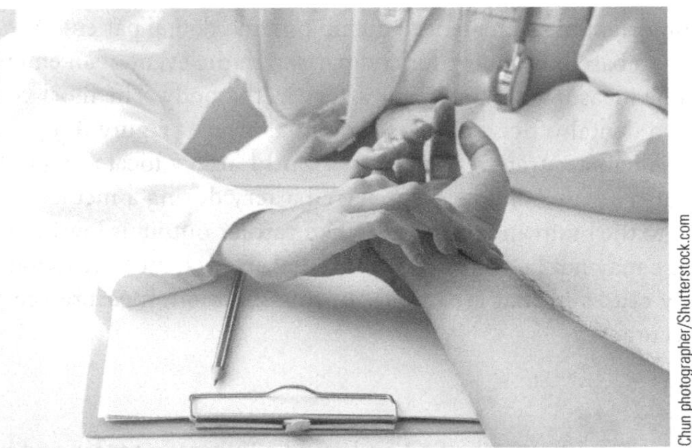

Chun photographer/Shutterstock.com

FIGURE 3-8 Recording pulse with the first and middle fingers

with a high pulse rate should not be scheduled for elective dental care until the cause of the elevated pulse rate is determined and brought to a safe level.

Measuring Radial Pulse

- Assemble armamentarium: medical history form, watch with a second hand.
- Wash and dry hands.
- Greet patient and introduce self.
- Explain procedure and purpose to patient.
- Review medical history of patient.
- Rest patient's arm and hand on a support such as the armrest of the dental chair. Face palm upward.
- Operator places fingers properly on thumb side of wrist (Figure 3-8).
- Count pulse for at least 30 seconds and multiply number of pulses counted by 2. Count for at least 1 minute if irregular pulse (such as a skipped beat) is detected.
- Describe if pulse is normal, fast, or slow, irregular or regular.
- Record pulse on medical history form.

RESPIRATION

The measurement of respirations involves counting the number of times the patient breathes in and out in one minute. A normal **respiration rate** range for an adult is 12–18 breaths per minute, although the rate can be dramatically different among certain groups of people, such as athletes. A faster than normal respiration rate is known as **tachypnea** and a lower than normal respiration rate is known as **bradypnea**. Tachypnea and bradypnea may be caused by disease processes. Tachypnea or bradypnea should be evaluated for causes prior to the start of dental treatment.

To measure the patient's respirations accurately, make sure the patient is unaware that you are watching them breathe. By the patient being unaware of your actions, you can record a more accurate respiration rate. If the patient is aware you are observing the respiration rate, there is a chance they may alter how they are breathing. Continue holding the patient's wrist as though you are still measuring the pulse while you actually watch and count the rise and fall of the chest. Respiration should be observed for a minimum of 30 seconds and then may be doubled for the 1-minute respiration rate. During cool weather when patients have on several layers of clothing, it is helpful to have the patient place one arm over the chest; the rise and fall of the arm then indicates the respirations.

Measuring Respiration

- Assemble armamentarium: medical history form.
- Greet patient and introduce self.
- Review medical history of patient.
- While patient is seated in the dental chair, count respirations while patient is unaware of this (Figure 3-9).

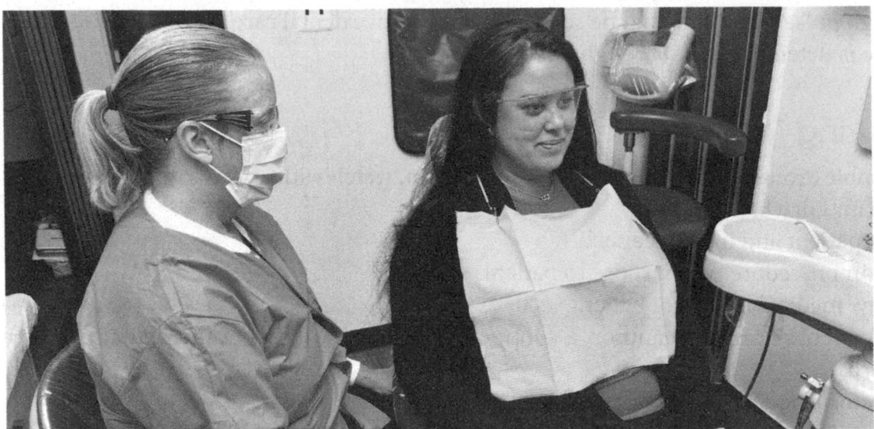

FIGURE 3-9 Counting respiration

- Count regular respirations for 30 seconds and multiply by 2. If an irregular respiration is noted, count respirations for one full minute.
- Describe respirations by depth and rhythm.
- Record respirations on patient's medical history form.

TEST YOUR KNOWLEDGE

1. What pulse site is used to measure pulse during an emergency situation?
2. Why do you record the respiration rate while the patient does not know you are observing it?

TEMPERATURE

A patient's body **temperature** is not usually measured in the dental office on a routine basis. However, if the dental team suspects that the patient may be ill, or if extensive surgery is to be performed, the dentist may request that the patient's body temperature be measured.

Use a thermometer to measure a patient's body temperature. Body temperatures vary throughout the day for each person and the average is 98.6 degrees Fahrenheit and ranges from 97 degrees Fahrenheit to 99 degrees Fahrenheit for an adult. Body temperature for a child of school age may range from 98 to 99. A variety of thermometers and methods for measuring temperature are available,

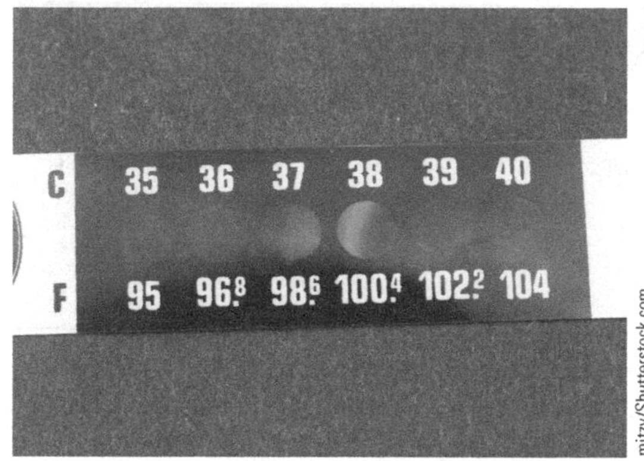

mitzy/Shutterstock.com

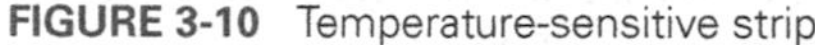

FIGURE 3-10 Temperature-sensitive strip

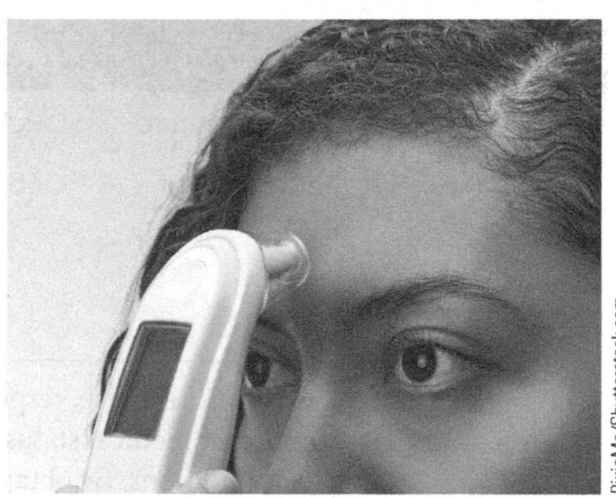

PixieMe/Shutterstock.com

FIGURE 3-11 Infrared Thermometer

including digital, temporal, tympanic thermometers, and temperature-sensitive strips (Figure 3-10). An oral digital thermometer is the type most often used in a dental office; however, non-contact infrared digital thermometers are increasingly popular (Figure 3-11). The dental staff should select an oral thermometer that best meets their needs. To prevent the transmission of bacteria from an ear or an oral thermometer, single use, disposable probe covers are recommended. The office may also choose to use a disposable thermometer.

Technique

The oral route is recommended for routine temperature measurement in the dental office. The technique described below is for use with an oral digital thermometer. If other methods are utilized, follow the manufacturer's instructions.

Measure Temperature

- Assemble armamentarium: medical history form, oral digital thermometer, appropriate barrier.
- Wash and dry hands and don gloves as well as protective clothing, mask and protective eyewear.
- Greet patient and introduce self.
- Explain procedure and purpose to patient.
- Review medical history of patient.
- Remove the thermometer from the storage container and place the appropriate barrier over it to prevent contamination.
- Confirm that the thermometer is activated.
- Place the thermometer sublingually in the patient's oral cavity.
- Instruct the patient to close their mouth and hold the thermometer in the mouth with their lips. Always caution the patient not to bite the thermometer.
- Remove the thermometer from the patient's oral cavity and record the reading.
- Clean the thermometer according to the manufacturer's instructions.

TABLE 3-2 Recording Vitals

Date	Blood Pressure	Pulse	Respiration	Temperature
2/1/2019	124/82 Right arm	65/minute	14/minute	97.5° Oral digital thermometer

SUMMARY

Vital signs such as blood pressure, pulse, respiration, and temperature are an excellent means of determining the patient's current medical status. In addition, the health history informs the dentist of past and present medical conditions. By obtaining all this information, the dentist and the auxiliary have taken the first step in assessing the patient's general health status. It is extremely important to have all vital signs accurately recorded in the patients chart for that day (Table 3-2).

REVIEW QUESTIONS

MULTIPLE CHOICE

1. Which of the following is/are considered a vital sign?
   a. temperature
   b. vision
   c. pulse
   d. both a and c

2. Which of the following are needed to record blood pressure?
   a. sphygmomanometer
   b. thermometer
   c. stopwatch
   d. all the above

3. Which artery is used to measure blood pressure?
   a. femoral
   b. carotid
   c. radial
   d. brachial

4. Respirations should be measured for ___ seconds.
   a. 30
   b. 15
   c. 10
   d. none of the above

5. Which of the following is not correct regarding obtaining baseline vital signs at the initial dental visit?
    a. Baseline vitals should be obtained at the first visit because the patient is less apprehensive at the initial visit.
    b. Baseline vital signs can help the staff respond during a medical emergency.
    c. Vital signs may vary depending on age, gender, weight, and physical health.
    d. It is not important to obtain baseline vital signs for dental treatment.
6. In addition to the four primary vital signs, height and weight can be recorded. Height and weight would be needed in pediatric dentistry to prescribe medications for the patient.

    Select the correct response based on the statement above.
    a. Both statements are true.
    b. Both statements are false.
    c. The first statement is true, the second statement is false.
    d. The first statement is false, the second statement is true.
7. Match each of the vital signs with the correct normal range.
    a. pulse
    b. blood pressure
    c. adult temperature
        1. 97–99
        2. <120/80
        3. 60–80
8. A rapid pulse is defined as which of the following?
    a. tachycardia
    b. bradycardia
    c. arrhythmia
    d. bradypnea
9. Bradypnea is a faster than normal respiration rate. Tachypnea is a slower than normal respiration rate.

    Select the correct response based on the statement above.
    a. Both statements are true.
    b. Both statements are false.
    c. The first statement is true, the second statement is false.
    d. The first statement is false, the second statement is true.
10. The systolic blood pressure is the pressure required for the left ventricle to pump the blood to the remaining vessels in the body. The diastolic blood pressure is the pressure of the heart muscle at rest while it is refilling with blood.

    Select the correct response based on the statement above
    a. Both statements are true.
    b. Both statements are false.
    c. The first statement is true, the second statement is false.
    d. The first statement is false, the second statement is true.

TRUE OR FALSE

_______ 1. A normal range for respirations is 60 to 72.

_______ 2. The thumb and first finger should be used to measure the pulse because they do not have a pulse of their own.

_______ 3. Blood pressure may be recorded through any type of clothing.

_______ 4. The first sound heard when taking blood pressure is the diastolic reading

_______ 5. Baseline vital signs are important to record as they can be used as a reference in the event of a medical emergency

_______ 6. The normal range for a pulse is 40–50 beats per minute

_______ 7. Weight may be a vital sign that is needed when prescribing medications for children

_______ 8. When recording blood pressure, it is not necessary to note the arm that the reading was obtained from

_______ 9. Normal blood pressure is 120/80

_______ 10. It is perfectly safe to treat patients with hypertension since the dental practitioner is just working in the oral cavity.

MEDICAL EMERGENCY!

CASE STUDY 3-1

A 55-year-old female patient presents with a positive medical history. She indicates that she is taking prescribed medication for hypertension. After reviewing the medical history, the dental auxiliary obtains the patient's vital signs. The vital signs are: BP 120/70 L arm sitting, pulse 60 bpm, resp 18 rpm, and temp 98.6 degrees.

Questions

1. Is the patient's blood pressure within normal range?

2. What additional information should be included with the blood pressure recording?

CASE STUDY 3-2

A 25-year-old male patient presents with a negative medical history. After reviewing the medical history, the dental auxiliary obtains the patient's vital signs. The vital signs are: BP 200/114 R arm sitting, pulse 90 bpm, resp 20 rpm, and temp 98.6 degrees.

Questions

1. What should the dental auxiliary do after recording these vital signs?

2. What medical condition could the patient have that they are not aware of?

SECTION TWO

Altered Consciousness Emergencies

This section deals with medical conditions that can result in the patient becoming disoriented, confused, dizzy, or losing consciousness, thereby resulting in a medical emergency.

CHAPTER 4

Syncope

LEARNING OUTCOMES

Upon completion of this chapter, the student will be able to:

- Use terms presented in the chapter
- Discuss the physiology of syncope
- List signs and symptoms of vasovagal syncope
- Choose the correct course of management for syncope
- Discuss the steps required to manage an episode of vasovagal syncope
- Describe how syncope can be prevented
- Identify the causes for postural hypotension
- Discuss the prevention of postural hypotension
- Explain the steps involved in managing postural hypotension
- Compare and contrast vasodepressor syncope and postural hypotension

KEY TERMS

nonpsychogenic
postural hypotension
presyncope
prodromal
psychogenic
supine position
sympathetic autonomic nervous system
syncope
tricyclic antidepressants
vasovagal syncope

INTRODUCTION

The most common medical emergency that may be experienced in the dental office is **syncope** (better known as the common faint), a loss of consciousness caused by a decrease in the blood flow to the brain. This condition has decreased over the past several years due to the implementation of the **supine position** during patient treatment (Figure 4-1).

Syncope is most often caused by some form of stress: physical, emotional, or both. The causes may be the result of a psychological reaction, known as **psychogenic (vasovagal syncope)** or a physiological reaction, known as **nonpsychogenic (postural hypotension)**. For this chapter, both the psychological causes and the physiological causes of syncope will be discussed as well as prevention and management.

VASOVAGAL SYNCOPE

Vasovagal syncope, or vasodepressor syncope, results when your involuntary nervous system, the **sympathetic autonomic nervous system** (SANS), malfunctions in response to a trigger such as stress. In a dental office, there are many psychogenic factors to produce stress in a patient. This can include fear, pain, emotional upset, and anxiety that can be specifically related to the dental office in the following ways:

- Most dental patients have some degree of fear about dental treatment. When this fear becomes overwhelming and unmanageable, it can become a psychogenic cause of syncope.
- All the modern advances have come close to making routine dentistry a painless experience. Even so, in some situations (e.g., inadequate anesthesia), pain may be experienced. This type of sudden pain may cause syncope.
- Unfortunately, dentists often have to inform patients of a poor prognosis. Bad news can sometimes trigger an emotional upset in a patient severe enough to cause syncope.

These triggers cause a reaction that results in a dilation of the vascular bed, resulting in a large amount of blood being pumped—mainly to the muscles of the arms and legs (the "fight-or-flight" syndrome). Since the patient remains stationary in the dental chair, this extra blood is not recirculated adequately to the heart and tends to pool in the arms and legs. This results in a deficiency of blood to the heart, and thus a lack of oxygenated blood being supplied to the brain. As a result of the brain's deprivation of adequate oxygen, a state of unconsciousness occurs.

Signs and Symptoms of Syncope

Syncope usually occurs while the patient is upright, not while in the supine position, because the supine position allows gravity to ensure a sufficient oxygen supply of blood flow to the brain (Figure 4-1). Syncope is a relatively slow-occurring problem, usually passing through two different stages, in each of which the patient exhibits distinctive signs and symptoms.

Presyncope, the first stage, precedes actual loss of consciousness. During this stage the patient exhibits some **prodromal** signs such as pale skin color and a cold sweat. The patient may complain of feeling hot, dizzy, or nauseated. Vital signs at this time show a slight decrease in blood pressure and a rapid increase in pulse. The decrease in blood pressure is due to the dilation of the vessels,

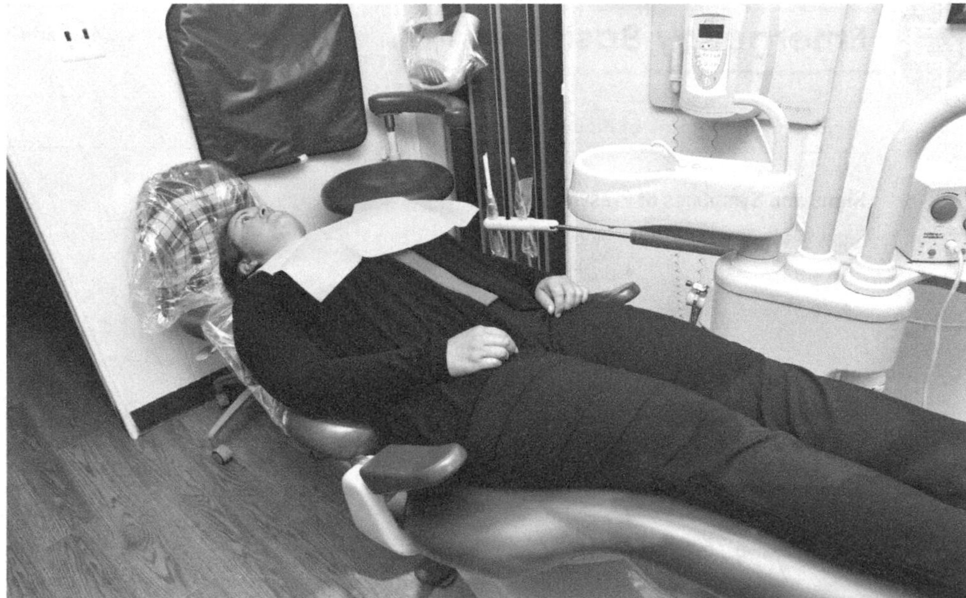

FIGURE 4-1 Supine position

and the increase in pulse rate is due to the heart pumping harder to send the blood to the brain. The heart can work this hard only for a short period of time. Once it tires, it no longer circulates a sufficient amount of blood. Therefore, the blood pressure and pulse rate drop rapidly immediately before the patient advances to the syncope stage. If the dental auxiliary identifies the prodromal signs of presyncope in a patient, they can prevent syncope from occurring.

Syncope, the next stage, consists of the actual loss of consciousness. During this stage, the patient exhibits a death-like appearance, the breathing may be shallow and gasping, slight convulsive movements may be present, pupils are dilated, and loss of bladder control may occur. Vital signs monitored at this time show a very low blood pressure and a slow, thready pulse.

See Emergency Basics 4-1 for a summary of the signs and symptoms of presyncope and syncope.

TEST YOUR KNOWLEDGE

1. Syncope caused by a psychological reaction is known as which type of syncope?

2. What is the primary cause of syncope in dental patients?

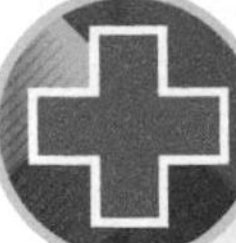

Emergency Basics 4-1

Signs and Symptoms of Presyncope and Syncope

Signs and Symptoms of Presyncope

Signs	Symptoms
• Pale	• Dizziness or lightheaded
• Cold sweat	• Nausea
	• Warm feeling
	• Tunnel vision

Signs of Syncope

- Death-like appearance
- Shallow, gasping breathing
- Dilated pupils
- Convulsive movements (possible)

Management of Syncope

First, remain calm. During syncope, as in all emergencies, the dental team must remain calm and in control. The patient who experiences syncope and revives to see a nervous and upset support group could very easily have a relapse.

As soon as the dental auxiliary suspects that a patient is experiencing syncope, stop all dental treatment. It was once believed to have the patient place their head between the knees. This is no longer accepted as a means of management. Placing the head between the knees makes it more difficult to breathe; in this position, the patient's brain does not receive adequate oxygen—which is what caused the episode in the first place. Instead, place the patient in the Trendelenburg position (Figure 4-2). Since most dental patients are already in the supine position, this position is easily achieved by slightly lowering the back of the chair. Placing the patient in this reclining position helps alleviate syncope because gravity is no longer a factor in getting blood to the brain.

If the patient loses consciousness in the waiting room or hallway, place the patient on the floor and elevate the legs slightly. This may be accomplished by placing an object such as a chair, coat, pillow, or a similar elevating device under the feet and legs. If nothing is available, simply hold the legs in an elevated position.

This positioning should be followed in every case when managing syncope except when dealing with a pregnant patient. If a pregnant patient is placed in the supine position, the weight of the fetus pressing against the diaphragm may inhibit breathing. Therefore, pregnant patients should be placed on their left side before elevating the feet.

Once properly positioned, the patient should recovery rapidly. If recovery does not occur right away, the next step is to make sure the patient has an open airway. When a person loses consciousness, the muscles of the tongue relax and the tongue may fall to the back of the throat, blocking the airway. When the airway is blocked, no oxygen goes to the brain, which could result in death. To open the airway, use the head tilt/chin lift techniques (see Figure 4-3).

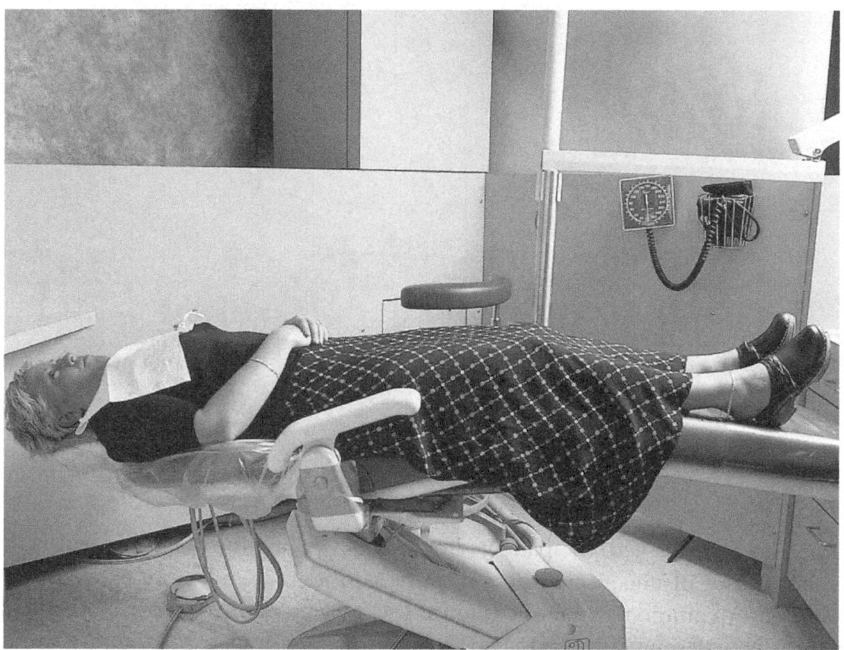

FIGURE 4-2 The Trendelenburg position is the most effective position in which to place a patient experiencing syncope because it uses the force of gravity to allow blood to flow to the brain
Source: Phinney/Halstead, Dental Assisting: A Comprehensive Approach 5e, Cengage, 2018.

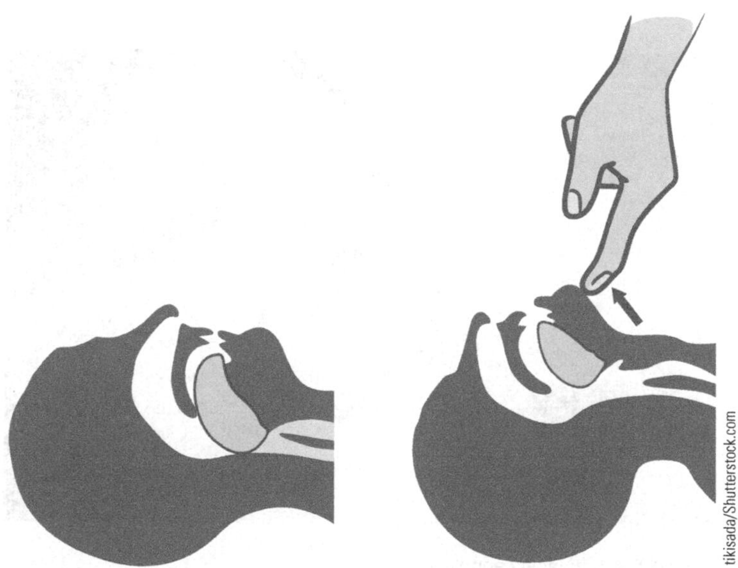

FIGURE 4-3 Chin tilt to open airway

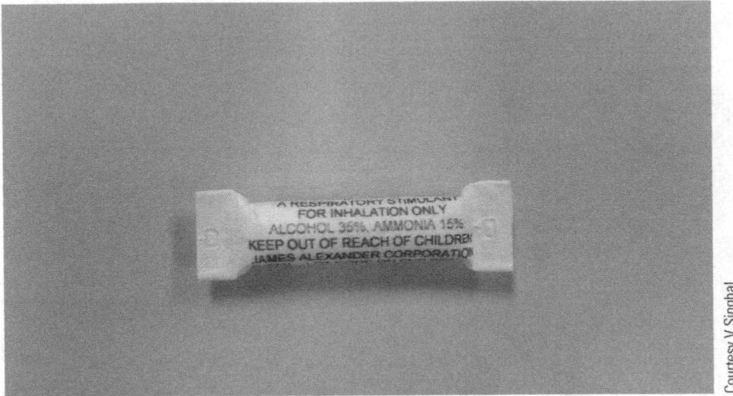

Courtesy V Singhal

FIGURE 4-4 Ammonia vaporole

After the airway is opened, the patient should begin to breathe on their own. If this does not happen, other causes of unconsciousness must be considered, and more extensive management may be required. An ammonia vaporole (Figure 4-4) may be cracked and passed quickly back and forth under the patient's nose for one to two seconds to help stimulate breathing. Ammonia gas will irritate the membranes of the nose and lungs, causing a reflex to initiate inhalation. The ammonia vaporole should never be left in place under the nose for an extended period of time, as it can irritate the nasal membranes and cause difficulty in breathing. Pure oxygen via a full face mask or a nasal cannula (Figure 4-5) also may be administered to aid in breathing and recovery. The vital signs should begin to return to their baseline readings during recovery.

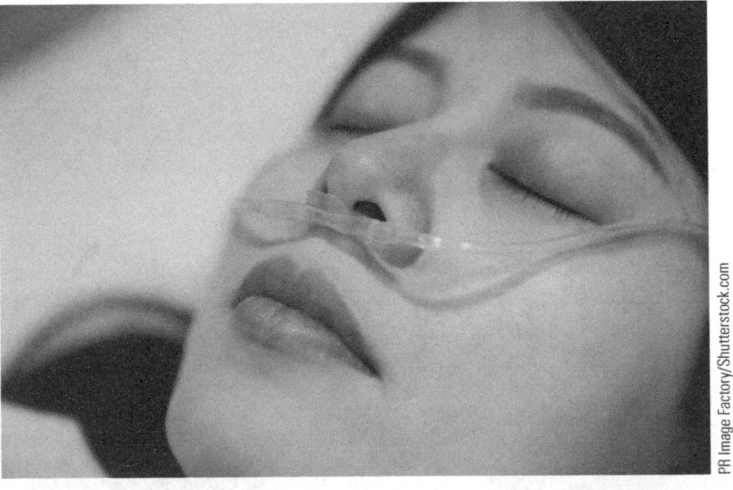

PR Image Factory/Shutterstock.com

FIGURE 4-5 Nasal cannula

Anything that can be done to help make the patient more comfortable during and following a syncope episode should be done. This could include placing a cold towel on the forehead or providing some type of covering if the patient complains of being cold once they begin to recover.

Recovery from a Syncopal Episode

On first recovering from an episode of syncope, a patient may be slightly confused and upset. The situation should be explained to the patient in a calm, reassuring manner. Some patients may be embarrassed by the episode; if so, extra efforts should be made to put the patient at ease.

A patient who has experienced a syncopial episode may faint again soon after recovery. Therefore, it is important to remove any predisposing stimuli such as needles and blood from the patient's sight. It is also important not to raise the patient too soon to prevent a second episode of syncope. Reschedule treatment for another day as recovery from vasovagal syncope may take several hours. Determine what led to the syncopal episode. Question the patient as to whether or not the syncope may have been caused by fear and/or anxiety during the procedure as well as regarding last meal eaten. Once the cause is determined, treatment modifications may be made for the next appointment. Modifications may include sedation with nitrous oxide and oxygen or an oral sedative.

Release the patient with a family member or friend once it has been determined that the syncopal episode was not caused by an underlying medical condition. It takes up to 24 hours for the vital signs to return to normal; thus, a patient who has experienced syncope should not be allowed to drive home. If the dentist believes that the episode was caused by a medical problem, EMS should be called and the patient taken to the hospital for further evaluation. EMS should also be called if the patient does not regain consciousness rapidly once they are positioned.

All the information concerning the episode should be documented in the patient's chart, including the signs and symptoms exhibited and the management provided. An example of management of syncope is outlined in Emergency Basics 4-2.

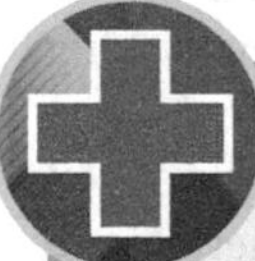

Emergency Basics 4-2

Management for Syncope

1. Remain calm
2. Place patient in Trendelenburg position (or if patient is pregnant, on their left side)
3. Maintain open airway by using head tilt chin lift method
4. Use ammonia capsule
5. Provide oxygen
6. Monitor vital signs
7. Make patient comfortable
8. Record all information in patient chart

TEST YOUR KNOWLEDGE

1. What position should the patient be placed in during a syncopial episode?

2. Why should treatment be rescheduled after a syncopal episode?

Prevention

Syncope may be prevented by maintaining a thorough, updated health history on each patient. Discuss with the patient any dental fears or any past negative experiences that may lead to stress and anxiety. The patient who has a history of syncope is more likely to experience it during a dental visit. If the staff should determine what causes that person to faint, extra precautions can be taken to prevent the patient from experiencing triggering conditions.

If the signs and symptoms of presyncope begin and are noticed early enough, in most instances, the operator can prevent the patient from advancing to the full syncope stage. When such signs and symptoms as cold sweat, nausea, or dizziness are present, stop dental treatment and place the patient in the Trendelenburg position. Also try to remove or alleviate whatever caused the patient distress in the first place. In most cases, patients will recover completely without experiencing syncope.

Furthermore, it is possible to prevent any signs and symptoms of any phase of syncope. Since fear and anxiety are the most common causes of syncope in the dental office, the easiest way to prevent syncope is to alleviate such fear and anxiety. This can be achieved by doing everything possible to make the patient comfortable, which may include talking with the patient; providing a bright, cheery atmosphere; and alleviating unpleasant sounds and smells associated with the dental office. In some cases, it might be helpful to premedicate a patient to alleviate extreme anxiety. Good local anesthesia technique is important in keeping the patient pain-free and comfortable during the dental procedure.

POSTURAL HYPOTENSION

Non-psychogenic syncope is known as postural or orthostatic hypotension. The cause of this syncope is significantly different than for loss of consciousness in vasovagal syncope. As discussed, vasovagal syncope has a psychogenic cause, and postural hypotension results in loss of consciousness that is caused by an underlying physiological problem.

Physiological Aspect of Postural Hypotension

Loss of consciousness due to postural hypotension occurs in patients undergoing a positional change from a prolonged supine position to an upright position. In some cases, a patient's body may not be able to adjust to the change in position, and the patient will suddenly lose consciousness. This occurs because gravity allows the blood to flow to the brain more readily when the patient is in the supine position. When the patient is placed upright, the blood vessels are unable to instantaneously constrict and blood pressure drops, eliciting unconsciousness.

One key difference between vasovagal syncope and postural hypotension is that there are no prodromal signs or symptoms in postural hypotension as there are in vasovagal syncope. Additionally, orthostatic hypotension occurs rapidly.

Predisposing Factors of Postural Hypotension

Predisposing factors in orthostatic hypotension are varied. Table 4-1 identifies predisposing factors to postural hypotension. A thorough medical history will reveal to the dental practitioner any conditions for the patient that could result in orthostatic hypotension. It is also important to question whether or not the patient has lost consciousness in the past.

TABLE 4-1 Predisposing Factors to Postural Hypotension

Elderly patients	Varicose veins may be one cause
Pregnant women, first or second trimester	Due to circulatory system expansion and a decrease in blood pressure
Pregnancy, third trimester	Caused by female lying supine for several minutes. Turning the patient to her left side will reduce the pressure on the vena cava and prevent loss of consciousness.
Heart conditions	Myocardial infarction, heart valve defects, or congestive heart failure can result in decreased blood pressure caused by poor circulation.
Medical conditions	Hypoglycemia in a patient with diabetes, hypothyroidism, adrenal insufficiency (Addison's disease) can result in a drop in blood pressure.
Many commonly used medications	Blood pressure medications, tricyclic antidepressants, antipsychotic medications, PDE5 inhibitors, sedative agents used in the dental office
Prolonged recumbence period such as long appointments	Move dental chair into upright position slowly to allow patient to adjust to change in position.

TABLE 4-2 Protocol for Prevention of Postural Hypotension

Return dental chair slowly to an upright position.

- From supine raise chair to a semi-supine position and allow patient to sit for 2 or 3 minutes.
- Raise chair to fully upright position and allow patient to sit for 2 minutes while the body adjusts.
- Allow patient to rise from chair slowly to a standing position. The practitioner should stand near the patient in case of loss of consciousness.

TABLE 4-3 Protocol for Managing an Episode of Postural Hypotension

- Assess situation and use head tilt, chin lift method to open the airway.
- Check for breathing.
- In supine position, the patient should recover quickly.
- Upon recovery, follow the protocol outlined in Table 4-2.
- If recovery is not immediate, a more serious underlying medical problem should be considered and EMS should be called.

Prevention of Postural Hypotension

Table 4-2 provides the steps the practitioner should implement to prevent an episode of postural hypotension. Table 4-3 provides the steps the practitioner should take in the event there is loss of consciousness due to an occurrence of postural hypotension.

If the cause of the loss of consciousness was postural hypotension and the patient has experienced loss of consciousness due to postural hypotension in the past, the appointment may proceed if both the practitioner and the patient see fit. At the end of the session, the patient may be dismissed without an escort because once the body has adjusted to the positional changes, a second syncopal episode is not likely to occur. However, if this syncopal episode has occurred for the first time, the patient should be dismissed with a family member. A physician should determine the cause of the syncope, and the dental appointment should be rescheduled.

DIFFERENTIAL DIAGNOSIS

Although the end result of both vasovagal syncope and postural hypotension is a loss of consciousness, the cause of both of these events is unique. Table 4-4 summarizes the differences between them so the operator is better able to manage loss of consciousness.

TABLE 4-4 Comparison of Vasovagal Syncope and Postural Hypotension

Characteristics	Vasovagal Syncope	Postural Hypotension
Prodromal signs and symptoms	Yes	No
Psychogenic cause	Yes	No
Fight-or-flight response	Yes	No
Caused by body's inability to adjust from supine to upright	No	Yes
Occurs rapidly	No	Yes
Dental appointment may continue if dentist and patient see fit	No	Yes if there is a past history

SUMMARY

By being familiar with the patient's history and taking extra effort to reduce stress in the dental office, the auxiliary can prevent most cases of syncope from occurring. However, in the event syncope does occur, the well-trained auxiliary can correct a potentially life-threatening emergency by following the basic management procedure of placing the patient in the correct position, maintaining an open airway, and administering ammonia and oxygen.

REVIEW QUESTIONS

MULTIPLE CHOICE

1. The main cause of syncope is
   a. hunger.
   b. stress.
   c. excitement.
   d. overactivity.

2. Which of the following conditions would be considered a psychogenic factor of syncope?
   (1) high blood pressure medication
   (2) fear
   (3) pain
   (4) poor health

a. 1, 2, 3
b. 1, 2
c. 2, 3
d. 3, 4

3. During which stage of vasovagal syncope would the patient complain of being dizzy and hot?
   a. syncope
   b. presyncope
   c. a and b
   d. none of the above

4. Which of the following are sign(s) of the syncope stage of vasovagal syncope?
   (1) cold sweat
   (2) nausea
   (3) dilated pupils
   (4) dizziness
   a. 2, 4
   b. 1, 3
   c. 3
   d. 1

5. Placing a patient in the supine position with the feet elevated is known as the __________ position.
   a. Trendelenburg
   b. prone
   c. recovery
   d. syncope

6. The purpose of the ammonia capsule is to
   a. burn the nasal passages.
   b. stimulate breathing.
   c. provide 100 percent oxygen.
   d. none of the above

7. Which of the following is correct regarding postural hypotension?
   a. It has a psychogenic cause.
   b. It occurs slowly.
   c. The patient exhibits prodromal signs and symptoms.
   d. It is caused by a rapid change in position from supine to upright.

8. Which of the following is correct regarding vasovagal syncope?
   a. Syncope is a loss of consciousness due to an increase in the flow of blood to the brain.
   b. Vasovagal syncope has no prodromal signs and symptoms

c. Vasovagal syncope progresses slowly as compared to postural hypotension
d. The cause of vasovagal syncope is usually physiologic and not psychogenic

9. When prodromal signs and symptoms are seen in a patient with a history of postural hypotension, immediately place the patient in the supine position to prevent loss of consciousness. When dismissing a patient with a history of postural hypotension, raise the chair from supine to upright in a slow manner to prevent loss of consciousness related to postural hypotension.

   Select the correct response based on the statements above.
   a. Both statements are true
   b. Both statements are false
   c. The first statement is true, the 2nd statement is false.
   d. The first statement is false, the 2nd statement is true.

10. Which of the following patient would be the least likely to experience loss of consciousness due to postural hypotension?
    a. Pregnant female in the 3rd trimester
    b. Patient with a history of myocardial infarction
    c. Patient taking blood pressure medications
    d. Healthy patient with no medical conditions

TRUE OR FALSE

_______ 1. Syncope is a life-threatening emergency.

_______ 2. Once a patient has experienced syncope, they are a likely candidate for it to recur.

_______ 3. Nonpsychogenic factors are the most common cause of syncope in the dental office.

_______ 4. Fear is an example of a psychogenic factor causing syncope.

_______ 5. During presyncope there is a decrease in blood pressure and an increase in pulse rate.

_______ 6. A good treatment for syncope is to have the patient place the head between the knees.

_______ 7. Since the patient is unconscious, it is not important for the dental team to remain calm while managing syncope.

_______ 8. If presyncope is recognized and managed properly, most instances of syncope can be prevented.

_______ 9. The patient may leave the office immediately after recovering from vasovagal syncope.

_______ 10. For orthostatic hypotension, a second syncopal episode is not likely to occur.

MEDICAL EMERGENCY!

CASE STUDY 4-1

A 32-year-old female presents with a positive medical history. She is six months' pregnant and has come to the dental office because she has had some pain in the maxillary right central. While waiting for the dentist to come into the operatory, she complains of feeling hot and a little dizzy. A few minutes later she loses consciousness. The auxiliary assumes the patient is suffering from syncope. She places the patient in the supine position, administers oxygen, and passes an ammonia capsule underneath the patient's nose.

Questions

1. What should the auxiliary have done when the patient first began to complain of feeling hot and dizzy?

2. Why should the patient not have been placed in the supine position?

3. What important treatment step did the auxiliary omit?

CASE STUDY 4-2

A 45-year-old male presents with pain in the maxillary right molar. He is taking a tricyclic antidepressant. He is otherwise in good general health, but he has not seen a dentist for 10 years. After the dentist completes treatment, the dental auxiliary sits the patient upright. Upon sitting the patient upright, the patient loses consciousness.

Questions

1. What condition is the patient most likely experiencing?
2. What is most likely the cause of this episode?
3. What should the dental auxiliary do first?
4. What could have been done to prevent this experience?

CHAPTER 5

Seizure Disorders

LEARNING OUTCOMES

Upon completion of this chapter, the student will be able to:

- Define epilepsy
- Explain possible causes of epilepsy
- Distinguish the phases of a tonic-clonic (grand mal) seizure
- Define an absence (petit mal) seizure
- Identify types of seizures based on a sign that is occurring
- Categorize the different seizures by onset
- Differentiate between status epilepticus and a non-static seizure
- Explain how epileptic seizures may be prevented
- Discuss the management of an epileptic seizure
- Describe some possible dental implications of epilepsy

KEY TERMS

absence (petit mal) seizure
aura
biofilm
clonic
convulsion
Dilantin® gingival hyperplasia
Down syndrome
electrolyte
epilepsy
epileptic cry
febrile
gingival hyperplasia
idiopathic
Jacksonian seizure
partial (focal or localized) seizure
status epilepticus
tonic
tonic-clonic (grand mal) seizure

INTRODUCTION

Nearly 3 million Americans, of all ages, suffer from seizures. A seizure occurs as a result of a sudden discharge of electrical energy somewhere in the central nervous system caused by an imbalance among the neurons of the brain. A seizure is also known as a fit or **convulsion**. The area of the brain that is affected determines the type of seizure the patient experiences. **Epilepsy** is a type of seizure disorder that affects people for a variety of reasons and is not selective as to ethnicity, age, or gender. The incidence of epilepsy is highest in those under the age of 2 and over the age of 65.

A seizure is a single occurrence, whereas epilepsy is more than one seizure that is unprovoked. For instance, temporary problems such as drug use, high fever, or abnormal glucose levels may be the cause of some seizures, which usually does not occur again once the cause has been corrected. Since these seizures occur only once, the patient does not have epilepsy.

CAUSES

Approximately 70 percent of cases of epilepsy are **idiopathic** in nature. Despite the fact that most cases have an unknown cause, certain triggers, such as flashing lights, will cause a seizure in those with the disorder. For the remaining 30 percent of cases, the cause is usually identifiable. It has been documented that if both parents have epilepsy, the chances of their children or descendants developing a seizure disorder are greatly increased. Table 5-1 provides predisposing factors of epilepsy.

TYPES OF SEIZURES

Seizures are usually identified by the actions that occur while the seizure is in progress. The onset of the seizure is now classified as generalized, focal, and unknown. Generalized seizures effect both

TABLE 5-1 Predisposing Factors to Epilepsy

- Trauma to the brain
- Genetics
- Diagnosis of Down syndrome
- Brain tumors
- Electrolyte and metabolic imbalances can lead to seizures, but be reversed by treating the condition
- Certain medications
- In newborns, a lack of oxygen during childbirth or maternal drug use
- Alzheimer's disease is the most common cause in the elderly
- Stroke and head trauma
- Febrile seizures
- Hypoglycemia
- Local anesthetic overdose in the dental office

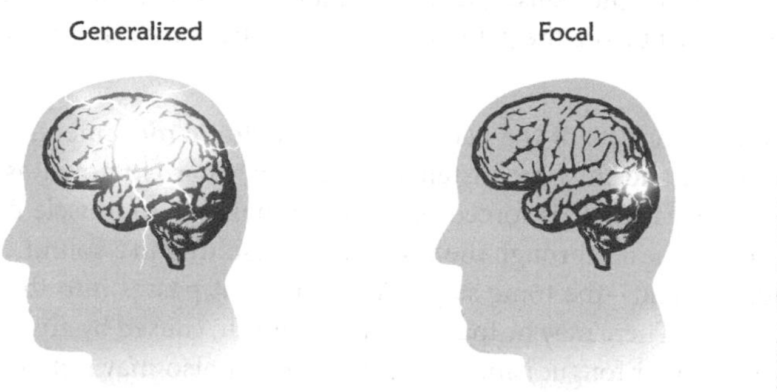

FIGURE 5-1 Generalized seizures versus focal seizures.

sides of the brain, focal seizures effect one side (Figure 5-1), and unknown simply means at the time the onset is unknown (such as when the person is found during or after the seizure). For unknown seizures, the onset is usually identified later. **Status epilepticus**, a life-threatening emergency, will also be discussed in this chapter.

Generalized Tonic-Clonic (Grand Mal) Seizure

The generalized **tonic-clonic (grand mal) seizures** are the most common. The term *tonic-clonic* is often used in place of *grand mal* in reference to the body movements the patient makes during the seizure. The generalized tonic-clonic seizure (GTCS) can be divided into three phases: prodromal, convulsive, and postictal (Figure 5-2).

Prodromal phase

The first phase is the prodromal phase, (aura phase) which includes the period before the actual seizure occurs. During this period, the patient may experience slight personality changes. These

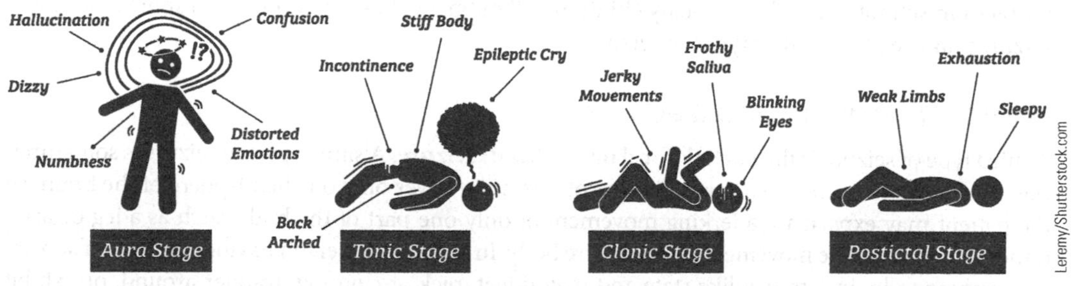

FIGURE 5-2 Stages of a generalized tonic-clonic seizure

are usually so subtle that they are noticed only by people who are very close to the patient, such as family members. Some patients may experience an **aura** during this phase. The aura may consist of a certain smell, a flash of light, nausea, déjà vu, or a certain noise. Auras are usually unique to the individual and occur just before the patient advances to the convulsive phase.

Convulsive phase

The convulsive phase consists of the actual ***tonic*** and ***clonic*** movements. The patient loses consciousness, falls down, and in some instances gives out what is known as an **epileptic cry**. The epileptic cry occurs because air is forced out of the lungs due to muscle contractions that occur. The contraction forces the air through the vocal cords, resulting in a sound. Next, the patient's body stiffens and becomes rigid—the tonic stage. As the patient passes into the clonic stage, the body begins to jerk violently. There may be foaming at the mouth, caused by air mixing with blood (if the patient bites their cheek or tongue) and saliva. The patient also may not be able to control bladder or sphincter muscles.

Postictal phase

The final phase of the grand mal seizure consists of the postictal phase. During this phase, the actual seizure is over, and the brain begins to recover from the seizure. The patient should slowly begin to regain consciousness. The patient may be confused about what happened and about where they are. In addition, the patient may need to sleep for a while to recover. While it is typical to recover in minutes, it could take hours or even days to fully recover.

Absence (Petit Mal) Seizure

Another type of seizure is the **absence (petit mal) seizure**. This type of seizure is not as common as the generalized tonic clonic seizure, about 200,000 cases occurring per year. The term *absence seizure* is used because it best describes what occurs during the seizure. Absence seizures can be typical or atypical.

The patient experiencing typical absence seizures will lose awareness of their surroundings for a short time. They may have a blank stare and can be mistaken for daydreaming, with some eye flutters (Figure 5-3). These seizures are usually short, only lasting about 10 seconds or so. This type of seizure can come and go without anyone around the patient realizing that they are experiencing a seizure. Atypical absence seizures will last longer, about 20 seconds. This type of seizure will start the same way with the addition of rapid eye blinking, smacking of the lips, and hand motions. Both types of absence seizures are most often seen in children and are often misdiagnosed as a behavioral problem in school-age children. Many children will outgrow these seizures but in some cases these seizures may lead into other types of seizures.

Partial (Focal or Localized) Seizure

A third type of seizure is the **partial (focal or localized) seizure**. A simple partial seizure is sometimes classified as a **Jacksonian seizure**. This type of seizure involves only one hemisphere of the brain, so the patient may experience a jerking movement of only one part of the body, such as a leg or arm, rather than convulsive movements of the entire body. In addition, a person having this type of seizure may appear to be in a trance-like state and may fidget, pick at clothing, wander around, or exhibit continuous lip smacking. In some cases, a partial seizure may progress into a full tonic-clonic seizure.

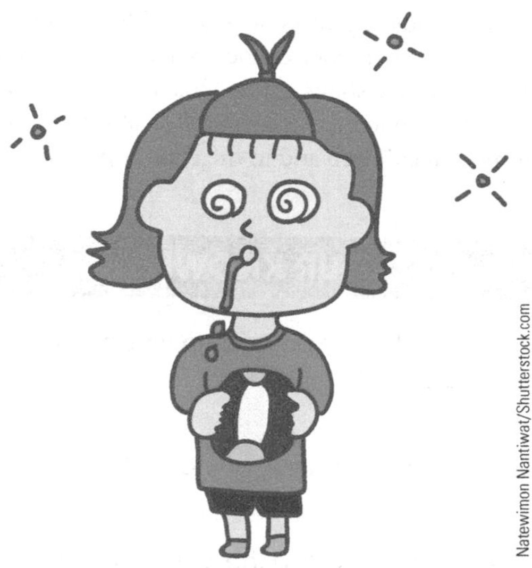

FIGURE 5-3 Absence seizure

TEST YOUR KNOWLEDGE

1. What type of seizure begins on both sides of the brain?

2. In what phase would a patient experience an aura?

3. Why do patients experiencing a seizure produce an "epileptic cry"?

Status Epilepticus

Status epilepticus is when a seizure lasts more than 5 minutes, or multiple seizures occur one right after the other, without giving the brain a chance to recover. In most situations, the longer the seizure lasts, the more likely medication will be needed to arrest it. Status epilepticus can be convulsive and non-convulsive. Any seizure can become a static seizure. However, the static GTCS can be life threatening. Medical management of a static seizure includes administration of intravenous anticonvulsive agents such as diazepam (Valium) or midazolam. Status epilepticus usually occurs in patients who are noncompliant with medications to control seizures or who have other underlying medical disorders such as brain tumors. Illicit drug use can also cause grand mal status seizures.

Rapid treatment by a trained medical professional is vital for status epilepticus. Non-convulsive status epilepticus involves a prolonged absence or focal seizure. The person is not unconscious but may appear confused. People at risk for status epilepticus are those with low blood sugar, uncontrolled epilepsy, and stroke. Status epilepticus accounts for about 10 percent of deaths related to epilepsy, and it is more common in children and in the elderly population.

TEST YOUR KNOWLEDGE

1. What condition is a patient experiencing when several epileptic seizures occur one after the other?
2. What type of seizure involves only one hemisphere of the brain?
3. What type of seizure may result in the patient having tonic and clonic movements?

PREVENTION

Most of the causes of seizures are still unknown, and in these circumstances it is impossible to prevent people from developing seizure disorders. However, in the majority of cases, seizure disorders can be controlled and seizures prevented through the administration of an anticonvulsant. One commonly used medication to control epilepsy is Dilantin, which will be discussed later in this chapter. An anticonvulsant medication cannot cure a seizure disorder, but it can control the seizures in about 75 percent of patients.

A thorough medical history will aid the dental professional in the identification of the patient with a history of seizures. Table 5-2 provides medical history questions related to seizures or epilepsy that the dental professional should ask a patient. Stress reduction protocol is important in preventing a seizure from occurring in the dental office. Stress reduction protocol is outlined in Table 5-3.

TABLE 5-2 Medical History Questions Related to Seizures and Epilepsy

- Returning patients should be questioned about recent hospitalization and any changes in medical history.
- Those with a history of seizures should be asked about the type of seizures experienced and what triggers a seizure. Some patients are well controlled due to the medications, and others may continue to experience seizures despite medications. A medical consult should be obtained from the treating physician prior to dental treatment of a patient who continues to experience seizures despite treatment.

TABLE 5-2 *(Continued)*

- Patients with a history of seizures should be questioned about their aura so the practitioner is aware a seizure may be forthcoming.
- Ask about how long the seizures last and any hospitalizations related to the condition.
- Note how often the patient sees the physician for management as well as the physician's phone number in the patient chart.
- Question the patient about medications used to control the seizures. Dilantin, valproic acid, carbamezapine, ethosuximide, and phenobarbital are some common medications a patient may be taking to manage epilepsy.

TABLE 5-3 Stress Reduction Protocol

- Premedication for anxiety if needed
- Morning appointments with minimal wait times are best
- Appointment length is determined by anxiety level and/or physical ability to tolerate longer appointments
- Nitrous oxide sedation as needed
- Good pain control methods during and after procedure as needed
- Follow-up phone call to patient later in the same day

If a seizure takes place in the dental office, try to recall what happened before the seizure occurred, as this may help you determine what triggered the episode. For example, was a material being used that had a distinct odor, or did an instrument emit a particular sound? By making this determination, it may be possible to prevent some seizures from occurring in the dental office in the future.

Stressful situations can trigger seizures in patients with a history of epilepsy. To many people the dental office provides just this type of situation. It is, therefore, extremely important to try to eliminate as much stress as possible. Ways to achieve this include:

- Show and demonstrate the use of all equipment in the office.
- Do not keep the patient waiting in the reception area for a prolonged period of time. This can result in anxiety that can trigger a seizure in those who have a history of epilepsy.
- In some cases, premedicating the patient with an antianxiety medication may be beneficial in preventing a seizure. This step requires a consultation with the patient's physician or neurologist.

DENTAL MANAGEMENT

Even with the best practices for prevention, the time may arise when a patient experiences a seizure while in care of the dental professional. It is important to be aware of how to manage an epileptic seizure should it occur in the dental office. Witnessing an epileptic seizure can be traumatic. When treating a patient experiencing a seizure, try to stay calm and remember that the seizure is usually brief and not life-threatening.

The dental professional's goal is to prevent the patient from injuring themselves during the actual seizure and to provide supportive help once the seizure is over. Emergency Basics 5-1 outlines the steps in management of a generalized tonic-clonic seizure.

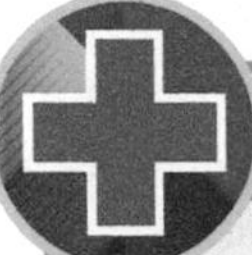

Emergency Basics 5-1

Grand Mal Seizure

1. If the practitioner is made aware of the aura and if time allows, remove all objects from the patient's oral cavity, move all objects from the treatment area to prevent harm to the patient, and move the patient to the floor. If the seizure begins without prior warning, it may not be possible to move the patient to the floor. Instead, lower the chair and place the patient supine.
2. Summon emergency medical services (EMS).
3. Time the seizure so you are aware of how long it lasts. This information can then be given to EMS once they arrive.
4. Maintain a patent airway with the head-tilt, chin lift method.
5. Use soft suction tips in the mucobuccal fold only to suction the airway of blood and saliva. **Do not** place anything between the teeth of the patient's maxilla and mandible as this can result in fractured teeth.
6. Gently restrain the patient only to prevent injury. Gentle restraining is only to prevent significant movement of the arms and legs that may result in injury. Protect the patient's head by placing a soft blanket or pillow or towel underneath if the patient is on the floor.
7. Monitor and record vital signs.
8. Upon termination of the seizure, prepare to manage the postictal phase. During this phase, the patient will sleep and should be placed in a supine position. Respiratory, cardiovascular, and central nervous system depression also occur during the postictal phase.
9. Oxygen may be administered to the patient and the airway should be maintained with the head tilt chin lift method. Monitor and record vital signs. The patient may take up to 2 hours to recover. Some patients go into a deep sleep for several hours. The patient should be given plenty of time to rest and recover in an appropriate area.
10. A determination must be made to discharge the patient to a hospital or send the patient home with a friend or family member. Only release the patient to go home once vitals have returned to normal and it has been confirmed that the patient is not confused or disoriented. If in doubt, EMS will transport the patient to a hospital.
11. In the event that the GTCS does not terminate within 5 minutes, it should be considered a grand mal status epilepticus seizure and managed aggressively. For the practitioner unfamiliar with administering IV anticonvulsants, the patient should be maintained until EMS arrives. Upon administration of IV anticonvulsant medications, the seizure will terminate. In all cases of grand mal status, the patient must be transported by EMS to a hospital for further management and evaluation.

Emergency Basics 5-2 summarizes these steps for the management of a patient having an absence seizure.

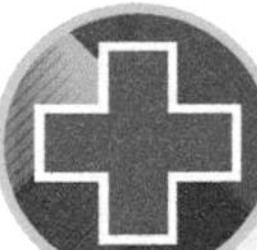

Emergency Basics 5-2

Management of an Absence Seizure

1. Minimal intervention is required as the seizure usually last for less than 30 seconds and seizure may be unnoticed at times.
2. If noticed by the operator and if time allows, prevent injury to the patient by terminating dental treatment and removing all objects from the patient's oral cavity and from the treatment area.
3. Offer reassurance and remain with the patient until the seizure terminates.
4. Dental treatment may continue if the patient and practitioner believe that it is appropriate to do so.
5. Determine what may have triggered the seizure so modifications may be implemented for future treatment.
6. If the seizure does not terminate within 5 minutes, EMS should be summoned and BLS implemented as necessary.

TEST YOUR KNOWLEDGE

1. What management would not be indicated for a patient experiencing a seizure?
2. Why should the dental professional not place any objects between the patient's teeth during a seizure?
3. How can the dental health care provider protect the patient's head during a generalized tonic-clonic seizure?

DENTAL IMPLICATIONS OF SEIZURE DISORDERS

The dental office is a likely setting for the occurrence of an epileptic seizure, just as it is for many other stress-related emergencies. Furthermore, the dental office may have to deal with special situations related to epilepsy or other seizure disorders.

The medications used to manage epilepsy are central nervous system depressants. As a result, patients may experience drowsiness. Some of the medications cause stomach upset and xerostomia as a side effect. As a result of reduced salivary flow, the patient may be more prone to decay and

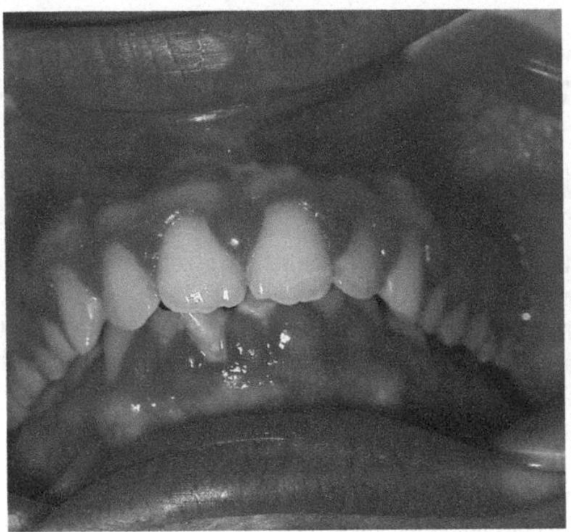

FIGURE 5-4 Dilantin gingival hyperplasia is a side effect of the commonly prescribed seizure disorder drug Dilantin

therefore should be educated regarding management of xerostomia. In addition, many patients will suck on candy or drink sugar-containing beverages to relieve the symptoms of xerostomia, increasing the risk of caries. Patients should be advised to use sugar free gum or candy and drink water. Saliva substitutes such as Moi-Stir or Xero-Lube may also be recommended.

Phenytoin, or Dilantin® is one of the drugs commonly given to treat seizure disorders. Patients taking this medication may produce a condition known as **Dilantin® gingival hyperplasia**, in which the gingival tissue grows at a rapid rate in an exaggerated response to **biofilm** and in some cases covers the teeth completely. Meticulous care at home is advised to help prevent further growth of the gingiva. In extreme cases, the tissue is surgically removed. Figure 5-4 demonstrates the effect of Dilantin® on a patient's gingival tissue.

TEST YOUR KNOWLEDGE

1. What anticonvulsant medication causes gingival hyperplasia?
2. What are the common side effects of epilepsy medications?

SUMMARY

Seizure disorders are mysterious, sometimes unknown origin, and can be frightening for both the patient and dental professional. However, by being prepared with a thorough review of the patient's medical history, understanding the stages of seizures and how to recognize them, and knowing how to manage a seizure should it occur can help reduce the risk of injury to the patient and the team.

REVIEW QUESTIONS

MULTIPLE CHOICE

1. If a person experiences several epileptic seizures occurring one after the other, what is the person most likely experiencing?
   a. an absence seizure
   b. status epilepticus
   c. a partial seizure
   d. none of the above
2. In most cases epilepsy can be controlled by administering what type of medication?
   a. antidepressant
   b. anticonvulsant
   c. antibiotic
   d. all of the above
3. What is an adverse dental condition that affects the gingival soft tissues and sometimes occurs as a result of taking Dilantin?
   a. hyperplasia
   b. xerostomia
   c. loss of taste
   d. loss of smell
4. Which of the following is not appropriate in the management of an epileptic seizure?
   (1) Loosen any tight clothing.
   (2) Restrain the patient from making any movements.
   (3) Remove any dental objects from the patient's oral cavity.
   (4) Do not move the patient unless it is absolutely necessary.
   a. 2
   b. 3, 4
   c. 1, 2, 3, 4
   d. 4
5. Which of the following may cause a person to develop a seizure disorder?
   a. injury to the brain
   b. eating healthy
   c. exercise
   d. no family history of epilepsy

6. During which phase of the grand mal seizure would the tonic/clonic movements be seen?
   a. prodromal
   b. convulsive
   c. postictal
   d. none of the above

7. During what type of seizure would the patient exhibit a blank stare and twitch or blink?
   a. grand mal
   b. status epilepticus
   c. partial
   d. absence

8. If a person experiences an aura, it usually occurs during which phase?
   a. postictal
   b. prodromal
   c. convulsive
   d. none of the above

9. Medical assistance should be summoned during which of the instances below?
   a. Status epilepticus is suspected.
   b. The patient is injured.
   c. The patient stops breathing.
   d. All the above

10. An absence or petit mal seizure is most often seen in which of the following?
    a. young adults
    b. children
    c. elderly
    d. teenagers

TRUE OR FALSE

_______ 1. All causes of epilepsy are unknown.

_______ 2. A patient should not be aggressively restrained during a seizure.

_______ 3. The most common type of seizure in children is a partial seizure.

_______ 4. The primary goal in treating an epileptic seizure is to prevent injury to the patient.

_______ 5. Anticonvulsants are not successful in treating most cases of epilepsy.

________ 6. Status epilepticus causes death in 10 percent of cases.

________ 7. Tonic/clonic movements are usually seen in absence (petit mal) seizures.

________ 8. It is acceptable to place a soft suction between the patient's teeth during a generalized tonic clonic seizure.

________ 9. Absence seizures are the most common type of seizure.

________ 10. Every epileptic experiences the same type of aura.

MEDICAL EMERGENCY!

CASE STUDY 5-1

A 32-year-old female presents with a positive medical history. She indicates that she has seizures that are not controlled with medication. The patient is scheduled for an initial examination. The dentist has become involved in an extensive procedure, and the patient is kept waiting in the operatory. During this time, she becomes very anxious about the upcoming treatment. The dentist enters the operatory and begins treatment. The patient is quiet and starts to twitch. She then proceeds to a full tonic-clonic seizure.

Questions

1. What could have been done that might have prevented the patient from experiencing the seizure?

2. How would being aware that the patient has a seizure disorder help during management of the episode?

3. Describe the signs this patient would exhibit that would indicate the seizure was a grand mal type.

4. Explain the management that would be provided for this patient.

CASE STUDY 5-2

A 29-year-old male patient presents with a positive medical history. He indicates that he has a seizure disorder but has been stabilized with medications and has not had a seizure in 18 months. The dental auxiliary enters the treatment room and begins speaking to the patient about the procedure on tooth #2. As the treatment explanation continues, the patient becomes more quiet and less responsive. The auxiliary notifies the dentist of the patient's change in consciousness.

Questions

1. What type of seizure is the patient experiencing?
2. How would knowing the patient's medical history help the auxiliary know what the patient is experiencing?
3. List the steps of the management that would be provided for a patient experiencing an absence seizure.

CHAPTER 6

Diabetes Mellitus

LEARNING OUTCOMES

Upon completion of this chapter, the student will be able to:

- Define diabetes mellitus
- Explain the function of insulin
- Compare and contrast type 1 and type 2 diabetes
- Explain two possible causes of diabetes
- Define oral hypoglycemics
- Define hyperglycemia
- List the signs and symptoms of hyperglycemia
- Describe the management of hyperglycemia
- Define hypoglycemia
- Describe the signs and symptoms of hypoglycemia
- Describe the management of hypoglycemia
- Describe the purpose of glucagon
- Differentiate between diabetic coma and insulin shock
- Identify two medical problems associated with diabetes
- Describe one dental problem with which the diabetic patient may present

KEY TERMS

diabetic coma
gestational diabetes
glucagon
glucose
HbA1C
hyperglycemia
insulin
insulin shock
ketones
macrovascular disease
microvascular disease
neuropathy
oral hypoglycemics
pancreas
periodontal disease
polydipsia
polyphagia
polyuria
subcutaneous

INTRODUCTION

The term *diabetes mellitus* came from Greek and Latin sources. Diabetes is translated as "run through a siphon"; *mellitus* means "honey." Together they are said to mean "sweet water siphon." The name *diabetes mellitus* was given to this disease because medical people of ancient times observed that persons with diabetes urinated frequently and their urine tasted very sweet. Today diabetes mellitus is defined as a metabolic disorder that occurs as a result of either an insufficiency or a complete lack of **insulin** (a hormone produced by the **pancreas**) in the body.

Diabetes mellitus is certainly not a new disease; it has been reported since Roman times. However, not until the early 1920s was a lack or absence of insulin discovered to be the cause of diabetes. Around 1921, insulin from animal sources began to be used in the management of diabetes. Beginning in the 1980s, technological advances resulted in the production of bioengineered insulin in laboratory settings. Currently it is this type of insulin that is prescribed by physicians for use by patients with diabetes.

FUNCTIONS OF GLUCOSE AND INSULIN

Glucose is the fuel for the body that is produced from the food we eat. Most of the cells in the body need glucose to survive. Glucose is carried to all cells by the bloodstream. However, for glucose to be able to enter the cell and provide it with the needed fuel, insulin must be present. In addition, the cells must also have insulin receptors. Patients with diabetes who must take injectable insulin have the condition in which the pancreas is either not producing enough insulin or not making it at all. Patients with diabetes who do not have to take insulin have a condition in which the pancreas produces enough insulin or perhaps even too much. The problem is usually that either there are not enough insulin receptors or these receptors are defective or have a lack of sensitivity to the insulin. These patients usually take oral medications to lower their blood sugar. These medications will be discussed later in this chapter.

It is of utmost importance that the glucose in the blood be kept at appropriate levels. Although glucose is the only fuel for the brain, too much glucose can be toxic to many tissues. Too much glucose therefore has the potential to cause as many problems as too little glucose. An imbalance of glucose in the blood results in some complications associated with diabetes, such as **macrovascular disease**, **microvascular disease**, and **neuropathy**. The imbalance of glucose also results in one of two conditions: hypoglycemia or **hyperglycemia**. Both imbalances will be discussed later in this chapter.

CLASSIFICATION OF DIABETES

Diabetes is classified as either type 1 or type 2. Type 1 diabetes was once known as "insulin dependent diabetes mellitus" (IDDM) or "juvenile diabetes" because it usually occurs in the young. The name was changed because the condition, although not common, has occurred in older people. A type 1 diabetic is insulin-dependent, which means the person must administer injectable insulin on a dosage prescribed by the physician. Insulin can be administered by daily **subcutaneous** injections (Figures 6-1a and 6-1b) or through an insulin pump (Figure 6-2). Insulin cannot be taken orally because it is a protein and would be digested by the stomach. Type 1 diabetes accounts for a smaller

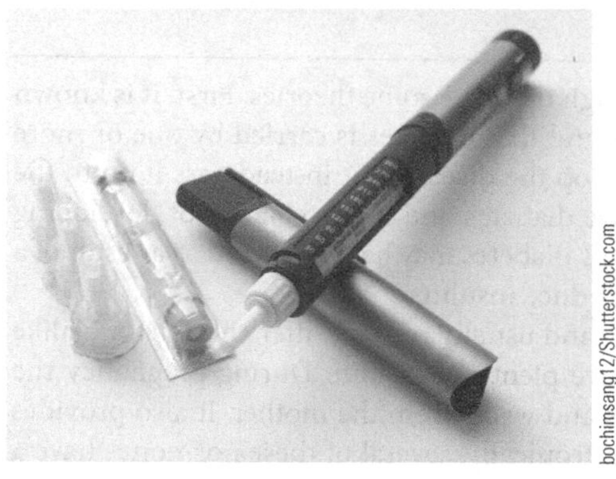

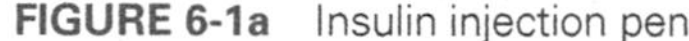

FIGURE 6-1a Insulin injection pen

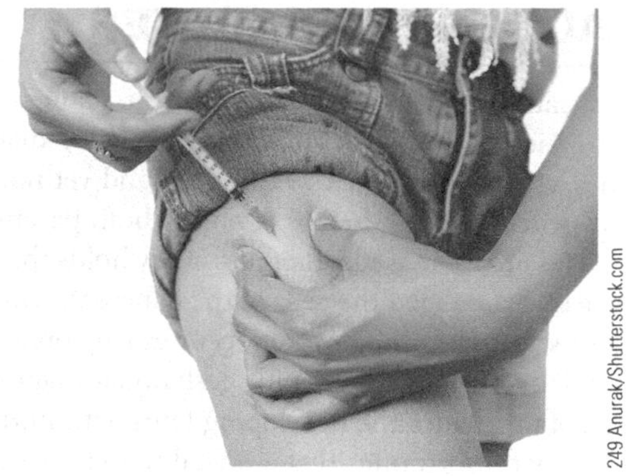

FIGURE 6-1b Subcutaneous injection of insulin

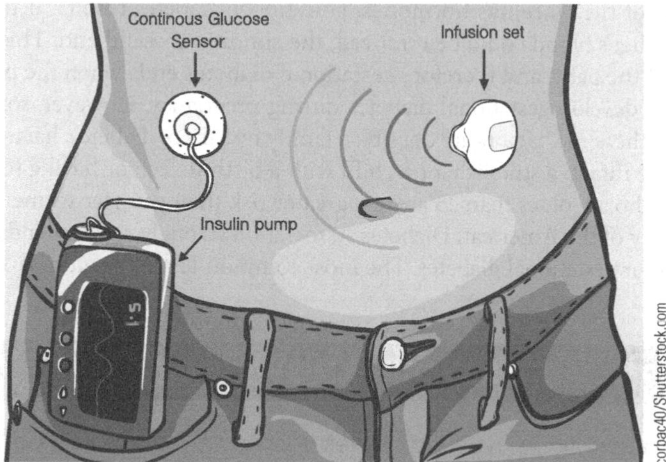

FIGURE 6-2 Administration of insulin through an insulin pump.

percentage of all cases of diabetes mellitus. The majority of the short-term and long-term medical problems associated with diabetes occur in type 1. Problems associated with type 1 diabetes will be discussed later in this chapter.

Type 2 diabetes has also been known as "adult-onset diabetes" or "non-insulin dependent diabetes mellitus (NIDDM)." Like type 1, this name was changed because this condition can also occur in the young. However, most people with type 2 diabetes are middle-aged and obese. Type 2 accounts for most of the known cases of diabetes. In most cases of type 2, injectable insulin is not required because the condition can usually be controlled with diet, exercise and medications known as **oral hypoglycemic**. These include drugs such as sulfonylureas, thiazolidinediones, alpha-glucosidase inhibitors, and metformin.

CAUSES OF DIABETES

Most causes of diabetes are idiopathic in nature, although there are some theories. First, it is known that genetics plays a definite role in causing diabetes and that diabetes is carried by one or more genes. A person may carry this gene and yet not develop the disease, but instead pass it on to the next generation. Therefore, if one or both parents have diabetes, the child's chances of developing diabetes are increased. Another theory holds that type 1 diabetes may have occurred as a result of a virus that damaged the cells of the pancreas, which produce insulin.

Gestational diabetes can occur during pregnancy and usually resolves after childbirth. Unlike type 1 diabetes, women with gestational diabetes have plenty of insulin. During pregnancy the placenta provides the developing fetus with nutrients and water from the mother. It also provides a variety of hormones that are vital to the pregnancy. Ironically, several of these hormones have a blocking effect on insulin. This blocking effect usually occurs approximately midway through the pregnancy. The larger the placenta becomes, the more blocking of the insulin occurs. This occurs in all pregnancies, and in most cases the woman can make additional insulin to overcome the blocking effect. However, when the pancreas makes all the insulin that it can and there still is not enough to overcome the effect of the placenta's hormones, gestational diabetes results. If the placenta's hormones from the mother's blood could be removed, the condition would end. This is what happens following delivery of the baby, and therefore gestational diabetes ends when the pregnancy ends.

Any woman may develop gestational diabetes during pregnancy. However, some women are at greater risk. Some of these risk factors are obesity; a family history of diabetes; having given birth previously to a very large infant, a stillbirth, or a child with a birth defect; or having too much amniotic fluid. Also, women who are older than 25 are at a greater risk than younger women. The Council on Diabetes in Pregnancy of the American Diabetes Association strongly recommends that all pregnant women be screened for gestational diabetes. The most common test is the glucose-screening test.

TEST YOUR KNOWLEDGE

1. What medication is type 1 diabetes treated with on a daily basis?
2. What medication is type 2 diabetes treated on a daily basis?
3. What is the cause of gestational diabetes?

ORAL HYPOGLYCEMICS

Oral hypoglycemics are medications that lower blood sugar. They are not effective in treating type 1 diabetes, in which there is no insulin production, but they have been found to be effective in some cases of type 2 diabetes. Most physicians suggest that it is best to treat type 2 with diet and exercise and, if medication is needed, to try oral medications. Oral hypoglycemics are not prescribed to pregnant patients or patients with liver or kidney problems.

DIABETIC EMERGENCIES: HYPERGLYCEMIA AND HYPOGLYCEMIA

The balance of glucose in the body must remain constant. If there is too much glucose, a condition known as hyperglycemia occurs. On the other hand, if there is too little sugar, a condition known as hypoglycemia occurs. Both conditions have the potential to develop into an emergency situation.

Hyperglycemia

Hyperglycemia occurs when there is too much glucose (sugar) in the blood and is usually seen when there is a deficiency or complete lack of insulin. Hyperglycemia is a slow-occurring condition. Because of the imbalance created in the cells, there is dehydration, which results in increased thirst and ultimately increased urination. Since the cells are not getting the energy that they need from glucose uptake, they are technically starving. As a result, the patient also exhibits hunger. These three classic signs of hyperglycemia are known as **polydipsia**, **polyuria**, and **polyphagia**. If the urine is checked, there will be a large amount of sugar and **ketones**. The ketones occur from the body fat breaking down for cell energy.

If hyperglycemia progresses without treatment, the patient may also exhibit loss of appetite, nausea and/or vomiting, fatigue, abdominal pains, and generalized aches. Additionally, the untreated hyperglycemic patient exhibits a heavy, labored breathing called Kussmaul breathing. The patient's breath has a fruity acetone odor as a result of the extra sugar. This is the condition present in the undiagnosed diabetic patient. Without treatment, this person will lose consciousness and go into what is called a **diabetic coma,** and possibly die.

Diabetic coma was the most common cause of death among people with diabetes in the years before the discovery of insulin. Today diabetic coma should rarely occur in known diabetic patients because symptoms of diabetes are diagnosed well before the coma occurs. Also, if the diabetic patient is testing their blood sugar on a regular basis using a glucometer (see Figure 6-3), the

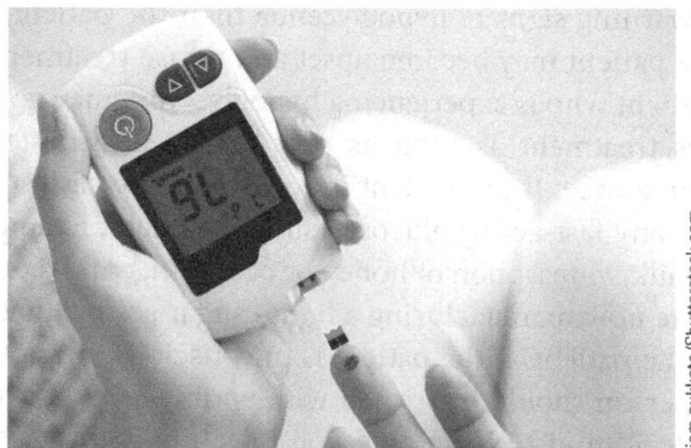
siam.pukkato/Shutterstock.com

FIGURE 6-3 A glucometer is a testing kit used by people with diabetes to measure the level of sugar in blood

patient will be able to identify problems before they advance into a diabetic coma. Diabetic coma can nevertheless cause death to patients with diabetes, especially patients with uncontrolled diabetes.

People who experience hyperglycemia require insulin injections; if conscious, they should administer their own insulin. Patients who are unconscious and experiencing a diabetic coma should be transported to a medical facility by the emergency medical service. The dental office is not equipped to manage hyperglycemia. The dental staff should never attempt to administer insulin to an unconscious patient because the amount of insulin required is not known.

Hypoglycemia

Hypoglycemia occurs as a result of too little glucose in the body. Since glucose is the only source of fuel for the brain, if the brain goes for a long time without adequate glucose, brain-cell damage may occur. Episodes of hypoglycemia are more common in a diabetic patient and are usually the diabetic emergency that will be more commonly seen in the dental office.

Hypoglycemia usually has a rapid onset and may be caused by any of the following situations:

- The diabetic patient may have taken their insulin and skipped a meal or not eaten the balanced diet their disease requires. As a result, the insulin level is too high and the glucose level too low. Important questions to ask patients who have diabetes prior to any dental treatment are when they ate their last meal and what they ate. The answers to these questions can help the dental auxiliary determine if a diabetic emergency is possible.
- The patient may have exercised intensely, which used the sugar sources within the body. Diabetic patients are encouraged to exercise. However, there must always be a constant balance among exercise, food, and insulin. Diabetic patients monitor their blood glucose levels with multiple checks throughout the day and night.
- A change in routine occurs, such as when a young person goes off to college. The new patterns, schedules, and emotional stress may all cause an imbalance in the insulin and glucose levels that may result in hypoglycemia.

A person exhibiting hypoglycemia may break out in a cold sweat and appear nervous, trembling, weak, and hungry. There is usually a personality change that may include irritability, confusion, and the inability to think clearly. Often a family member or close associate of the patient may be better able to detect warning signs of hypoglycemia than the patient, since the patient may be confused. Sometimes the patient may become upset and refuse treatment as a result of confusion. An untreated diabetic patient who is experiencing hypoglycemia may go into **insulin shock**.

This patient requires treatment as soon as possible. Treatment for hypoglycemia includes administration of a sugar source. If the patient is conscious, the easiest method is to give a glass of orange juice, although any fast-acting glucose source will help. Examples of fast-acting glucose sources are 8 ounces of milk, ½ teaspoon of honey or cake icing, and 4 ounces of regular (not diet) soda. Some companies are now manufacturing a liquid sugar source that is available in a tube and is easy to administer to the patient. If the patient is unconscious, do not attempt to give anything by mouth. Instead, the person should be treated with an injection of **glucagon** if available and if the dentist is comfortable administering a glucagon injection. Glucagon is a hormone, produced in the pancreas, that raises blood sugar. It achieves this effect by changing the sugar stored in the liver into a source of sugar that can be used by the body. As soon as hypoglycemia is diagnosed in the unconscious patient, an injection of glucagon should be given. Once the patient regains full consciousness, orange juice should be administered. Glucagon is used up quickly, and if another source of sugar is not given, the patient may relapse into hypoglycemia. A second option is to administer intravenous glucose if the dentist is comfortable starting an IV. Remember that only drugs that the dentist and staff are comfortable administering should be included in the dental emergency kit. Alternatively, in the dental office, cake icing should available and can be applied to the mucobuccal fold. The sugar from the cake icing will be absorbed rapidly in the body, resulting in a reversal of the hypoglycemia. The patient should regain consciousness if the loss of consciousness was caused by hypoglycemia.

See Emergency Basics 6-1 for management of an episode of hypoglycemia.

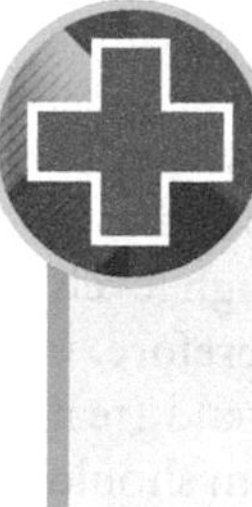

Emergency Basics 6-1

Management of Hypoglycemia (Insulin Shock)

Conscious patient	• In the conscious patient, a sugar source such as glucose tablets, chocolate, orange juice, apple juice, or a non-diet soda may be administered. • Upon ingestion of the sugar source, the signs of hypoglycemia reverse rapidly. In many cases, the patient will have a sugar source with them. • If a sugar source is not administered, the patient may lose consciousness.
Unconscious patient	• A glucose injection or an IV glucose solution may be administered. In case an IV is not practical, cake icing may be placed in the mucobuccal fold of the patient. The sugar from the icing will be absorbed slowly through the oral mucosa and recovery may take up to 30 minutes. The patient should be monitored at all times and a patent airway should be maintained. DO NOT ADMINISTER JUICE OR SODA TO THE UNCONSCIOUS DIABETIC PATIENT.

Diabetic Coma or Insulin Shock?

If the dental team finds a diabetic patient unconscious, it will be hard to determine whether the patient is experiencing a diabetic coma, insulin shock, or a related medical problem. If the dental team knows from the patient's medical history that the patient has type 2 diabetes and does not self-administer insulin, they may infer that the patient is experiencing a diabetic coma

TEST YOUR KNOWLEDGE

1. What are the noticeable signs and symptoms of hypoglycemia?
2. What can occur if the patient is not treated for hypoglycemia?

and should receive immediate medical attention. If the team members have no idea what type of diabetes the patient has, then they should treat the condition as insulin shock. It is important to get glucose into the system before the brain is damaged. An individual can withstand high levels of blood sugar much longer than the brain can survive with low levels of glucose. Therefore, if the dental team does not know which condition the patient is experiencing, they should treat for insulin shock. Once this treatment is performed, if recovery does not occur, the team should summon medical help.

CHRONIC MEDICAL PROBLEMS RELATED TO DIABETES

In addition to hypoglycemia and hyperglycemia, diabetic patients also have an increased risk of other medical problems. Diabetes increases the risk of macrovascular and microvascular abnormalities. These problems are mostly seen in the type 1 diabetic patient, particularly those who are poorly controlled.

Large-vessel problems are caused by the following:

- Inadequate blood supply to the heart muscle, resulting in conditions such as myocardial infarction or angina pectoris
- Inadequate blood supply to the brain, resulting in various types of cerebrovascular accidents (refer to Chapter 7)
- Inadequate blood supply to the legs, which increases the risk of infection, tissue necrosis, and amputations
- Inadequate blood supply to the kidneys, which results in kidney dysfunction or failure

Small-vessel problems most often affect the small vessels of the eye. This causes a disease known as diabetic retinopathy. This disease can cause blindness in patients with diabetes.

ORAL MANIFESTATIONS OF DIABETES

The diabetic dental patient can present with some unique concerns for the dental office. First there is a possibility that the patient may experience diabetic coma or insulin shock while in the office—the emotional stress of experiencing a dental procedure may be enough to exacerbate an already unstable situation. Additionally, if the patient is experiencing a particular medical problem associated with diabetes, such as high blood pressure or cardiovascular disease, the dental team may have to alter treatment to avoid an emergency situation.

The diabetic patient may experience some specific dental problems. For example, **periodontal disease** is extremely common in patients with diabetes. Furthermore, the periodontal disease tends to be more involved and more difficult to manage no matter how well the patient maintains good oral home care. There have been situations in which severe periodontal disease has caused a person's diabetes to become uncontrolled due to the level of infection and inflammation. Thus, it is important to keep the periodontal disease well controlled through regular office visits and good oral home care.

Patients with diabetes may experience delayed healing and as a result are more prone to infection. This is due to the circulatory problems associated with macrovascular and microvascular disease. The dental team, therefore, needs to be careful and cause as little tissue trauma as possible during dental procedures. Furthermore, if dental surgery is performed, frequent follow-up visits should be scheduled to ensure the patient is healing properly.

When treating a dental patient with diabetes, the dental team should ensure the following:

- Maintain a current, thorough medical history. It is important to realize the patient has diabetes. It is also important to know whether the patient is type 1 or type 2 and if the condition is controlled or uncontrolled at the time of the dental appointment.
- Consult with the patient's physician before beginning any extensive treatment. If the treatment that is to be provided will interfere with maintaining a normal routine, the patient's physician may need to make some changes in the insulin dose. Treatment planning should account for the fact that the diabetic patient needs to take their insulin and eat regularly. As a result, long appointments should be avoided, and an extensive treatment plan may need to be broken into multiple visits. There may also be some underlying medical problems that require special treatment or medication. It may be necessary to evaluate the patient's last **HbA1C** to determine how well controlled the patient's disease has been.
- Use effective local anesthetic techniques to ensure the patient remains relaxed and comfortable during each treatment session.
- Avoid making appointments that would cause the patient to miss a scheduled meal. Keeping diabetes under control means maintaining a balance among food, insulin, and exercise. Scheduling an appointment during lunch, for example, may upset the insulin balance and perhaps cause the patient to experience insulin shock. It may be necessary to monitor the patient's blood glucose levels using the patient's glucometer, especially if an appointment has interfered with a scheduled meal or snack.

It is beneficial for the members of the dental team to familiarize themselves with characteristics associated with diabetes. This is extremely helpful when providing treatment to certain age groups and patients with diabetes. For example, children with diabetes are sometimes concerned about experiencing new situations such as a trip to the dental office because they feel the dental staff will not understand their diabetes and therefore will not know what to do if they have any problems. It is important for each member of the team to understand the disease not just to know how to treat an emergency but also to know how to talk to and work with the patient.

SUMMARY

The study and treatment of diabetes has been focused for only about 60 years; advancements are being made rather rapidly and have been remarkable. New methods of diagnosing, treating, and controlling diabetes have been discovered. The space program has resulted in several advancements in the treatment of diabetes. Hopefully, soon, advancements will be made that will mean the dental team may not have to deal with emergencies such as diabetic coma and insulin shock.

REVIEW QUESTIONS

MULTIPLE CHOICE

1. Type 1 diabetes is most often treated with daily injections of ________.
   a. glucagon
   b. insulin
   c. oral hypoglycemics
   d. glucose

2. Type 2 diabetes may sometimes be treated with ____________.
   a. oral hypoglycemics
   b. glucagon
   c. glucose
   d. none of the above

3. Which of the following are signs or symptoms of hyperglycemia?
   (1) increased thirst
   (2) Kussmaul breathing
   (3) confusion
   (4) increased urination
   a. 1, 2, 3, 4
   b. 1, 2, 3
   c. 1, 2, 4
   d. 2, 3, 4

4. A hypoglycemic patient experiences elevated sugar levels. A hypoglycemic patient who is conscious should be given orange juice.
   a. Both statements are true.
   b. Both statements are false.
   c. The first statement is true, the second statement is false.
   d. The first statement is false, the second statement is true.

5. Which of the following are not signs or symptoms of insulin shock?
   (1) rapid onset
   (2) cold sweat
   (3) confusion
   (4) increased thirst
   a. 1, 2
   b. 3, 4
   c. 1
   d. 4

6. What is one option to manage insulin shock in the unconscious patient?
   a. giving orange juice
   b. administering insulin injection
   c. administering oral hypoglycemics
   d. placing cake icing in the mucobuccal fold

7. What is one example of a microvascular disease in a diabetic patient?
   a. angina pectoris
   b. diabetic retinopathy
   c. kidney dysfunction
   d. cerebrovascular accident

8. What is the only fuel for the brain?
   a. glucose
   b. insulin
   c. glucagon
   d. orange juice

9. What is the correct treatment for managing the conscious patient suffering from insulin shock?
   a. administer a sugar source such as orange juice
   b. administer insulin
   c. administer a glucagon injection
   d. administer a diet soda

10. A dental patient with diabetes may be more prone to which of the following?
    a. decay
    b. periodontal disease
    c. malocclusion
    d. all the above

TRUE OR FALSE

_______ 1. Insulin may not be taken orally because it is digested by the stomach.

_______ 2. Most medical problems are associated with type 2 diabetes.

_______ 3. Glucagon is administered to a patient who is experiencing hyperglycemia.

_______ 4. Type 2 diabetes was once called juvenile diabetes.

_______ 5. Oral hypoglycemic are used to manage type 1 diabetes.

_______ 6. Type 2 diabetes accounts for the majority of the diagnosed cases of diabetes.

_______ 7. Hyperglycemia is an elevation of blood sugar.

_______ 8. Genetics plays an important part in the cause of diabetes.

_______ 9. Insulin is produced in the body by the pancreas.

_______ 10. The dental office is well equipped to manage hyperglycemia.

MEDICAL EMERGENCY!

CASE STUDY 6-1

A 35-year-old female presents with a positive medical history. She is type 1 diabetic. Her dental treatment for today is an amalgam restoration. The dental auxiliary reviews the medical history and finds that the patient is a type 1 diabetic taking daily injections of insulin. The patient rushes into the office slightly late for her appointment. She reports that she was in such a hurry that she did not get a chance to eat lunch, but she took her usual dose of insulin. As the appointment begins, she breaks out in a cold sweat and appears nervous. When the dentist questions her, she seems confused.

Questions

1. What condition is the patient most likely experiencing?

2. What should be done to treat this condition?

3. How might this situation have been avoided?

CASE STUDY 6-2

A 23-year-old female presents with a positive medical history. She reports a history of type 1 diabetes. The patient is scheduled for a crown preparation at 8 a.m. When the dental auxiliary reviews the medical history, the patient indicates that she has an insulin pump. As the treatment progresses, the dental auxiliary notices that the patient's skin has become cold and clammy, and when the patient is questioned, she appears to be very confused.

Questions

1. What type of diabetes does the patient have?

2. What condition is the patient most likely experiencing?

3. How could this episode have been avoided?

CHAPTER 7

Cerebrovascular Accident (CVA)

LEARNING OUTCOMES

Upon completion of this chapter, the student will be able to:

- Define cerebrovascular accident (CVA)
- Classify the types of CVA
- Summarize the predisposing factors of a CVA
- List the signs and symptoms of a CVA
- Discuss the medical history questions related to identifying a patient who is at risk for a CVA
- Describe dental management of a CVA patient in the dental office

KEY TERMS

aneurysm
aphasia
arteriosclerotic
ataxia
atherosclerosis
atrial fibrillation
cerebrovascular accident
embolism
fibrin
hemiparalysis
hemorrhagic
intracerebral
ischemic
magnetic resonance image
palliative
platelet
sickle cell anemia
subarachnoid
thrombosis

INTRODUCTION

A **cerebrovascular accident** (CVA) is also known as a stroke. It is defined as a specific neurological deficit that occurs suddenly as a result of vascular disease of a **hemorrhagic** or **ischemic** nature (Figure 7-1). Figure 7-2 shows a **magnetic resonance image** (MRI) of a CVA. Patients who suffer from a CVA may recover completely, or the CVA may be severe enough to cause permanent disability or death. The result depends on the type of stroke, the extent of damage to the brain, and how quickly the patient receives medical care.

TYPES OF CEREBROVASCULAR ACCIDENTS

Ischemic Stroke

Eighty-seven percent of strokes are ischemic strokes. This type of CVA occurs when a blockage in a blood vessel supplying an area of the brain is present. This may be due to arteriosclerotic fat buildup in the blood vessels (Figure 7-3). Ischemia may also be caused by a thrombus (**thrombosis**) or an embolus (**embolism**) that occludes the vessel. A thrombus is a blockage composed of **platelets** and **fibrin**. It forms in a vessel and remains there, resulting in occlusion and reduced blood flow. A

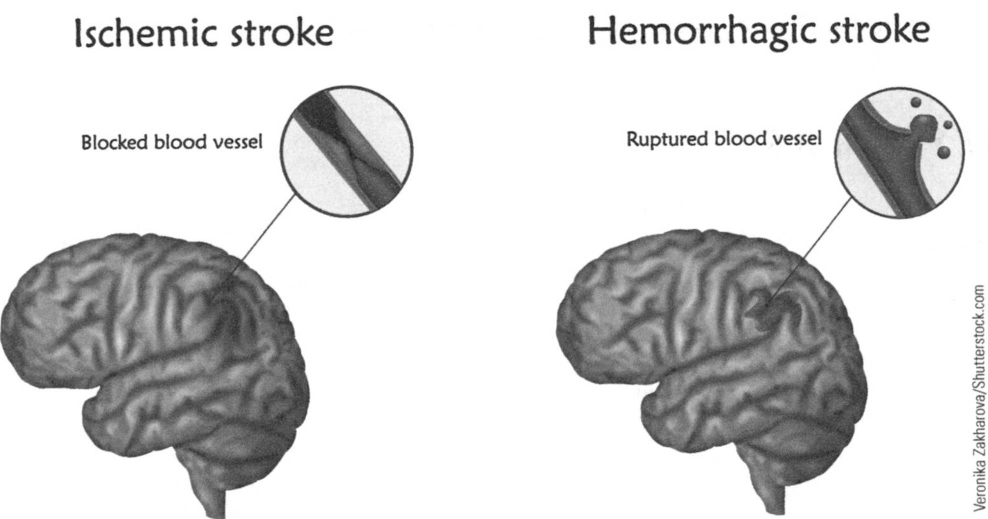

FIGURE 7-1 An ischemic stroke (left) happens when there is a sudden blockage, usually caused by a blood clot that deprives areas of the brain of proper oxygen. Ischemic strokes are the most common. A hemorrhagic stroke (right) is the rupturing of a blood vessel, resulting in a dramatic decrease in blood flow to the brain. An infarct is an area in the brain tissue that has died due to a lack of blood.

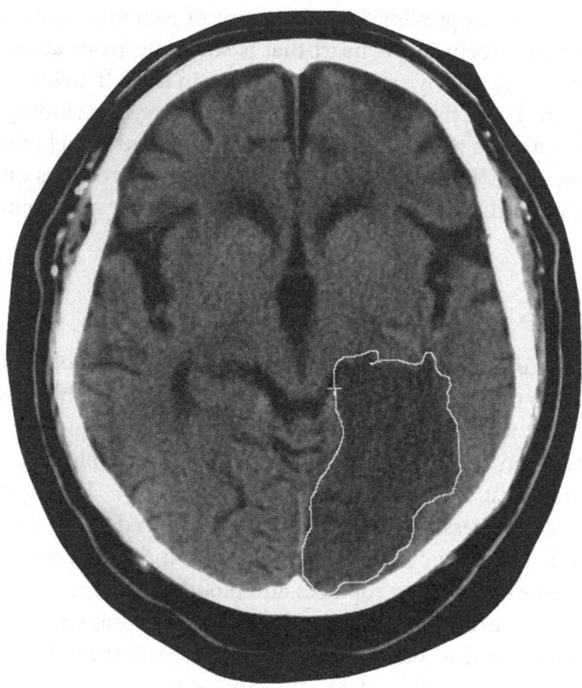

FIGURE 7-2 Magnetic resonance image of a brain with a visible bleed from a CVA in the lower-right section of the brain

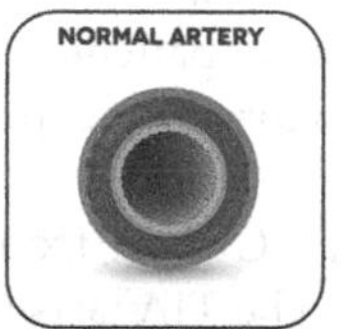

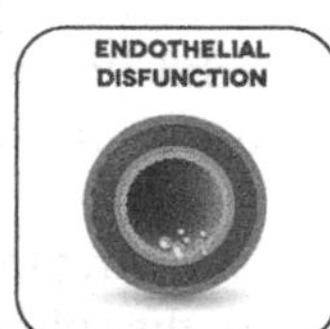

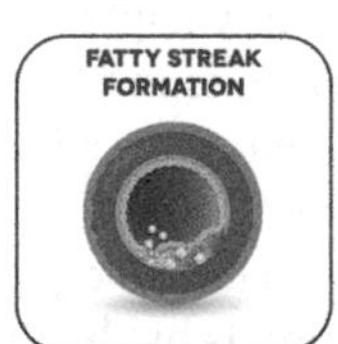

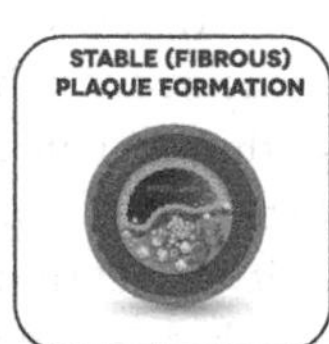

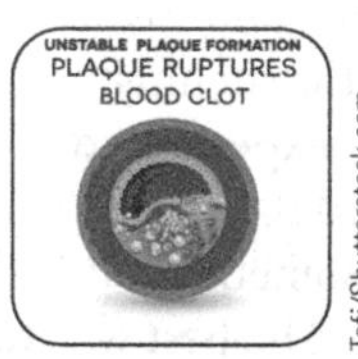

Tefi/Shutterstock.com

FIGURE 7-3 Progression of coronary artery disease, a risk factor for a cerebrovascular accident

thrombus begins when damage occurs to the lining of the blood vessel and the clotting process is initiated. Damage to the blood vessel lining occurs when plaque adheres to the walls of the vessels. Approximately 70 percent of ischemic strokes are the result of a thrombus.

An embolus is a clot that originated elsewhere in the body, usually in the larger vessels of the heart. Part of the clot breaks off and is now termed an embolus. It travels through the bloodstream and lodges in another blood vessel and causes an occlusion. If the embolus lodges in a vessel in the brain, the result may be a CVA. Approximately 30 percent of ischemic strokes are the result of an embolus. An embolus can also form in the heart that is suffering from **atrial fibrillation**. In this case, the atria do not contract effectively and the blood pools in the left atrium, causing an increased risk for thrombus formation. These thrombi can travel to other areas, including the brain, and lodge in a blood vessel. A third way that an embolus can lodge in a blood vessel in the brain is if the patient has a damaged heart valve. This can lead to formation of a thrombus on the damaged valve. The thrombus can break off and travel to a different part of the body as an embolus, including the brain.

Hemorrhagic Stroke

Hemorrhagic strokes make up approximately 13 percent of all cases of strokes. A hemorrhagic stroke occurs when an **aneurysm** ruptures. An aneurysm is an area of a blood vessel that has weakened and is ballooned out. If undiagnosed, it can continue to weaken until it ruptures. Hypertension may lead to a rupture. In the dental office, stress can elevate blood pressure and cause an undiagnosed aneurysm to burst, resulting in a hemorrhagic CVA. The rupture causes blood to enter the cranial cavity and put pressure on the brain, resulting in damage to the cells.

There are two types of hemorrhagic stroke: **subarachnoid** and **intracerebral**. In a subarachnoid stroke, a vessel on the surface of the brain ruptures and blood fills the space between the brain and the thin tissue that covers the surface of the brain. In an intracerebral stroke, a blood vessel within the brain ruptures, causing blood to damage the surrounding tissues. The intracerebral hemorrhagic stroke occurs more commonly than the subarachnoid type.

Transient Ischemic Attack (TIA)

A TIA is a neurologic deficit that lasts for a short period of time. Although a TIA is not an actual stroke, it is included in the classification of a CVA because it is so similar. A TIA is referred to as a warning stroke or a mini stroke. The relationship between a TIA and a CVA is similar to that of angina and myocardial infarction discussed in Chapter 11. Both are warning signs that a serious, life-threatening problem may occur. It has been found through careful questioning of patients who have experienced a stroke that they usually experienced some episodes of TIA before they experienced the complete cerebrovascular accident.

Sometimes it is difficult to determine whether the patient is suffering from a CVA or from a TIA. The best way to make that determination is by the duration of the episode. The TIA lasts less than a minute and then the signs and symptoms cease, whereas the signs and symptoms of a true CVA do not regress. The TIA is transient because the body was able to use its own clot-dissolving factors to dissolve the clot that was causing the blockage.

The clinical manifestations of a TIA vary according to the area of the brain affected. However, most people suffering from a TIA experience some numbness or weakness in the extremities. This numbness is sometimes described by the patient as a "pins-and-needles" feeling. Consciousness is usually not impaired, but the patient may appear somewhat confused during the episode.

The TIA does not usually present an emergency in the dental office. However, if the patient has a history of repeated TIAs, the dental team should realize that this patient has increased chances for experiencing a severe CVA, and treatment should be postponed until a medical consult can be obtained.

Always remember that a TIA has the potential to advance to a severe CVA. Whether a TIA advances to a complete stroke usually depends on the underlying cause of the TIA. If the cause is resolved, a CVA will not occur.

TEST YOUR KNOWLEDGE

1. What type of stroke is a result of a clot forming in some area of the body and traveling to the brain?
2. What type of stroke is most likely to occur in the dental office?
3. What type of stroke is a CVA with signs and symptoms that are exhibited for less than a minute?

PREDISPOSING FACTORS TO A CEREBROVASCULAR ACCIDENT

There are several predisposing factors that may lead to a CVA; some are modifiable, and some are not. Aging increases the risk for a CVA. After the age of 55, the risk of suffering from a stroke doubles for each decade of life. Race also is a predisposing factor. African Americans are at a higher risk for obesity, hypertension, and metabolic syndrome. As a result, this population is at a higher risk for a CVA as compared to Caucasians. The presence of family history also increases the risk for a CVA. Those who have suffered from a previous stroke are at a greater risk of suffering from a second CVA. People with a history of TIA are at higher risk for a stroke. Patients with **sickle cell anemia** suffer from a blood disorder in which the red blood cells are sickle shaped (see Figure 7-4). Because of the abnormal shape of the cell, they tend to stick to the walls of blood vessels. They can lodge in a cranial blood vessel and result in a CVA. All of the above factors are not modifiable.

Some predisposing factors can be modified or controlled, thus reducing the risk of a CVA. Hypertension is a predisposing factor that can be controlled through diet, exercise, and medications that can reduce the risk of a stroke. For patients who smoke, smoking cessation significantly reduces the risk of a CVA. When a person uses cigarettes and this is combined with oral contraceptives, the risk of a CVA significantly increases. All patients, including females using oral contraceptives, should be offered smoking cessation methods. Diabetes increases the risk of a CVA. Many diabetics

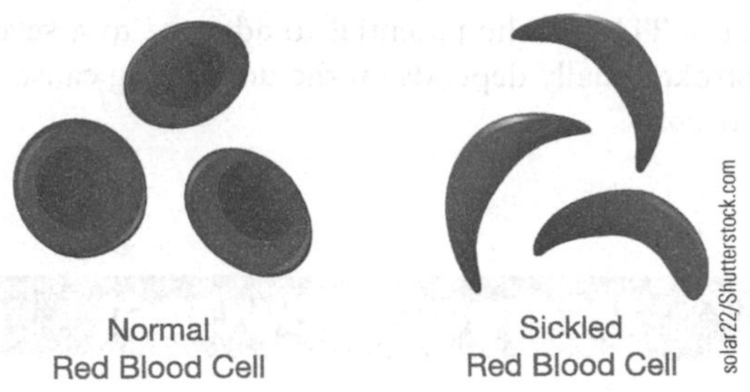

FIGURE 7-4 Comparison of a normal red blood cell to a sickled red blood cell

suffer from elevated cholesterol and hypertension, thus increasing the risk of a CVA even more. The well-controlled diabetic is less likely to suffer from systemic complications and vascular damage, thereby reducing the risk of a stroke. Patients with **arteriosclerotic** plaque buildup in arteries are at a greater risk for stroke as the plaque that is built up may dislodge and travel to lodge in a vessel in the brain. A healthy diet and increase in exercise help to reduce cholesterol levels, thus reducing plaque buildup in vessels. Lastly, a person who has a lack of activity is at higher risk due to inactivity leading to obesity, elevated cholesterol, and hypertension.

SIGNS AND SYMPTOMS OF A CEREBROVASCULAR ACCIDENT

Many of the signs and symptoms of a hemorrhagic stroke as compared to an ischemic stroke may be similar; however, there are some differences. A CVA caused by a thrombus is slow developing so in turn usually has a slow onset, whereas one caused by an embolus has a rapid onset. One common symptom of all CVAs is **hemiplegia** or paralysis on one side of the body. Paralysis will occur on the contralateral side (opposite side) of the cerebral infarct. Patients may also experience difficulty in speaking (**aphasia**) and difficulty in swallowing (**dysphagia**). CVA patients may also experience visual disturbances such as loss of vision or double vision. Patients suffering from a stroke often lose the ability of motor coordination resulting in **ataxia**. Other signs and symptoms include headaches, dizziness, numbness and weakness on one side of the body, and difficulty breathing. While loss of consciousness can be present in a hemorrhagic stroke, it is less likely to occur in an ischemic stroke.

A hemorrhagic stroke has a sudden onset. In addition to the above signs and symptoms, the hemorrhagic stroke can result in stiffness of the neck, nausea, and vomiting. The patient suffering from a hemorrhagic stroke will usually have hypertension at the time of the event because in most cases they are caused by elevated blood pressure. Loss of consciousness, should it occur, is a sign of a poor prognosis. The death rate of a hemorrhagic stroke is much higher than that of an ischemic stroke.

The American Red Cross teaches a mnemonic in its First Aid course that can be used to determine quickly whether a patient may be experiencing the signs and symptoms of a cerebrovascular accident. The mnemonic is FAST (Figure 7-5). See Emergency Basics 7-1 for more information on this mnemonic.

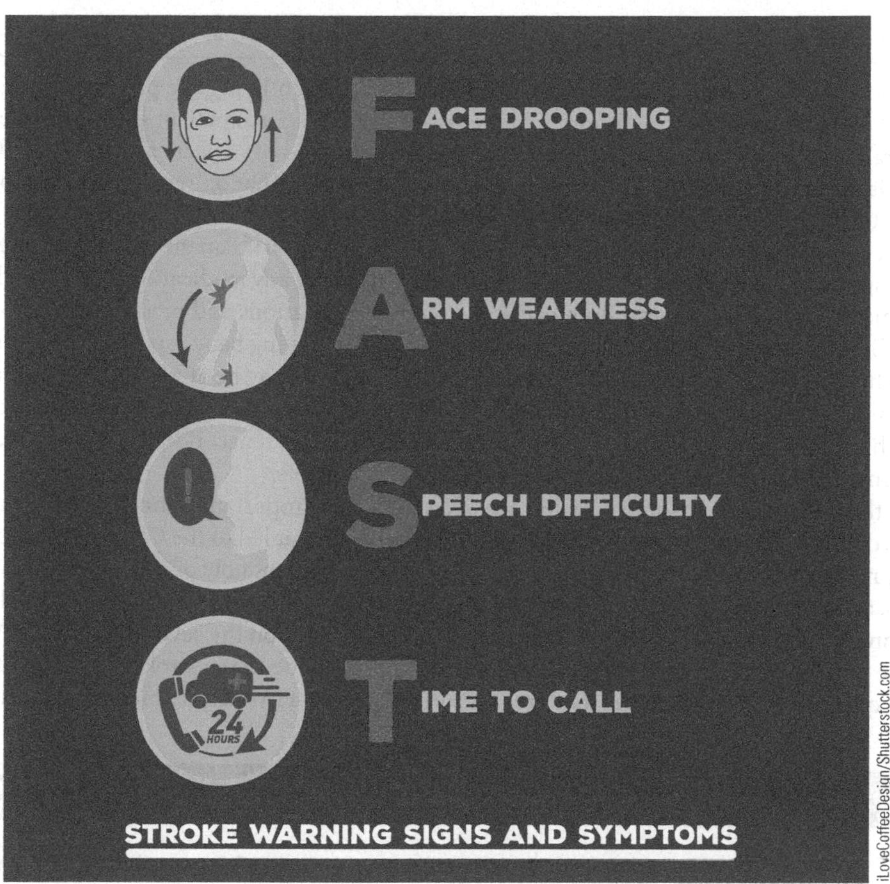

iLoveCoffeeDesign/Shutterstock.com

FIGURE 7-5

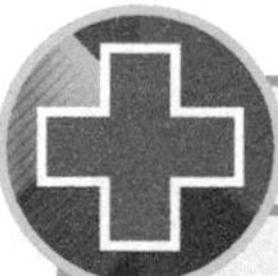

Emergency Basics 7-1

Recognizing a CVA: FAST

- **F = FACE** Ask the patient to smile. An asymmetry or drooping of one side of the face can indicate a potential stroke.
- **A = ARM** Ask the patient to lift both arms. A weakness of one arm or inability to raise an arm can indicate a potential stroke.
- **S = SPEECH** Ask the patient to repeat a simple statement. Evaluate both the patient's ability to respond correctly and the patient's speech pattern (e.g., whether the phrasing is correct and whether speech is slurred).
- **T = TIME** Notify the dentist and activate the emergency protocols in the office as quickly as possible. Noting the time and extent of the deficits can be helpful to the responding emergency personnel.

MEDICAL HISTORY AND PREVENTION

A thorough medical history will aid the dental auxiliary in identifying the patient who may have suffered from a stroke in the past or is at higher risk for a CVA. Each patient should be questioned on overall health changes as well as hospitalizations within the past 3 years as well as whether the patient is under medical care. If the patient is unsure of any information regarding health or medical events, the treating physician should be contacted.

Vital signs should be taken as a baseline and noted in the chart. Patients should be questioned regarding presence of hypertension. Question the patient about any medications and regarding any visual disturbances or dizziness. Both over-the-counter medications and prescription medications should be included in the discussion. Some patients may be taking baby aspirin daily to prevent a CVA. This should alert the dental practitioner that the patient may be at a higher risk for a stroke due to underlying predisposing factors. Post-CVA patients may also be taking baby aspirin or a blood thinner such as coumadin daily to prevent a second occurrence. If the stroke was caused by hypertension, the patient may also be taking an antihypertensive.

For the patient who has a positive history of a stroke, it is important to find out when the CVA occurred and what was the cause of it. If it was hypertension that led to the CVA, do they know the blood pressure reading at the time of the occurrence? Is the patient now on antihypertensive medications, and is the blood pressure now controlled? Are they compliant with taking this medication? How long the patient was hospitalized will provide information on the severity of the CVA. Question the patient on recovery from the damage that occurred due to the stroke. The patient should also be questioned about whether they are still suffering from TIAs despite medical intervention.

TEST YOUR KNOWLEDGE

1. What medical conditions on a patient's medical history indicate that the patient might have an increased risk of experiencing a CVA?
2. What are the general signs and symptoms of a CVA?
3. Which CVA has a rapid onset?

DENTAL MANAGEMENT OF A CVA PATIENT

Patients who have suffered from a CVA in the past six months are not candidates for elective dental care. The risk of a second stroke occurring is much higher during the six-month period following an incident. Patients may receive **palliative** care until the six months has passed. If treatment is necessary during the initial six-month time period, it should be performed in a hospital setting in case of the event of an emergency. After six months has passed, the patient may be treated after a medical consult. The dental team must be sure to implement stress reduction protocol and excellent pain management. This includes earlier appointments after the patient is well rested, shorter appointments, and local anesthetic that provides excellent pain control with no more than the cardiac dose of epinephrine. This would limit the local anesthetic to 2 cartridges of 1:100,000 epinephrine concentration or .04 mg of epinephrine. Stress, anxiety, and pain can trigger a CVA in a patient who is at risk for a CVA. Emergency Basics 7-2 reviews the ASA classifications of patients who suffered a CVA.

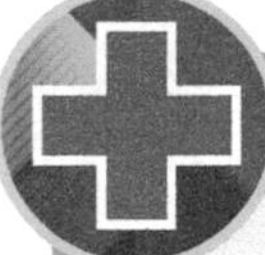

Emergency Basics 7-2

ASA Classification of a CVA Patient

- ASA II: The patient with no or very minor residual neurological effects
- ASA III: The patient with significantly impaired speech or impaired mobility which requires assistance
- ASA IV: The patient who has significant residual mental effects and may be immobile due to the severity of the CVA. This patient may also suffer from significant dysphagia or aphasia.

Since post-CVA patients are usually taking medications that interfere with platelet aggregation, bleeding may be prolonged. If the treatment plan includes invasive procedures that may result in bleeding, evaluation of bleeding time should be completed. The dentist can request blood test results that include bleeding time. If, after consult with the physician, it is determined that the patient may bleed excessively, several options may be considered. One of the options is the physician may choose to decrease the dosage of the antiplatelet medications for a period before the procedure to reduce platelet aggregation, thus reducing the bleeding time. Another option is the dentist may proceed with the treatment plan and be prepared to implement local methods such as sutures and cellulose sponges to enhance clotting and healing. Lastly, the dentist may opt to alter the treatment plan to minimize the risk of bleeding.

Implementation of stress reduction protocol is critical to minimizing the possibility of a CVA in patients at risk. Morning appointments are preferable as the patient has rested overnight. Appointments should be short, so extensive treatment plans should be divided into multiple visits. Use of the cardiac dose of epinephrine will allow adequate pain control and minimize stress caused by pain. Nitrous oxide sedation is also beneficial in minimizing a stroke in patients at risk. Patients who have elevated blood pressure post-CVA despite medical management are at high risk for a second incident. Patients considered to be high risk should not be treated electively.

MANAGEMENT OF A CVA IN THE DENTAL OFFICE

If a CVA occurs while the patient is in the dental office, the dental team should not waste time trying to determine the cause. The same emergency treatment is administered regardless of cause.

A dental team that recognizes the signs and symptoms of a CVA should be most concerned with monitoring the patient's respiratory and circulatory status. It is important to ensure the airway is open and adequate oxygen is available, since the patient is already suffering from an oxygen deficiency. See Emergency Basics 7-3 for management of a CVA in the dental office.

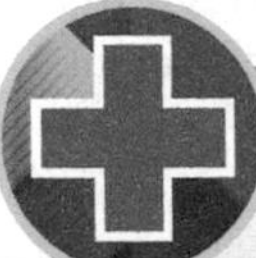

Emergency Basics 7-3

Protocol for Management of a CVA in the Dental Office

- Terminate dental treatment and remove all objects from the patient's oral cavity.
- Palpate carotid artery to assess circulation.
- Ensure that the patient has a patent airway and is breathing. In most cases, the patient will be able to maintain an airway without assistance.
- Position the patient in Fowler's position or semi-upright to reduce pressure on the brain and aid in minimizing damage (Figure 7-6).
- Monitor vital signs and record every 5 minutes. This information can then be provided to EMS. Keeping the patient calm is important. Summon EMS so patient can be transported to a hospital.
- Oxygen may be administered to the patient.
- It is important to not administer any sedative agents or other central nervous system depressants. These will mask symptoms and make diagnosis more difficult for EMS and the hospital staff.
- If the patient loses consciousness, the CVA may be extensive and time becomes critical for the patient. In the event of loss of consciousness, place the patient supine and perform basic life support (BLS) as needed. Once the patient has been transported to the hospital, more definitive care will be administered.
- In the event that the patient is suffering from a TIA, the symptoms should subside. It is best not to continue treatment at this time. The patient should be sent to a physician for evaluation. Treatment should resume once the patient has received medical care and after consult with the patient's treating physician. In most cases, the dentist should wait a minimum of six months before performing elective care procedures on the patient.

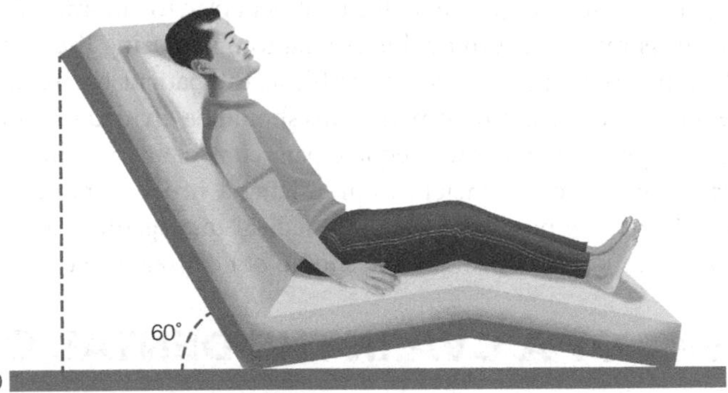

FIGURE 7-6 Fowler's position
Source: permobil

SUMMARY

Fortunately, a CVA is not a common occurrence in the dental office. Nevertheless, it can occur, and therefore the dental team must be prepared to treat such patients. As with all emergencies, the best treatment is prevention. The dental team can best achieve this by realizing that certain people are prone to CVAs. For example, diabetics, those suffering from hypertension, those with a history of cardiac disease, and those with a history of TIAs are more likely than other patients to experience a CVA in the dental office.

Furthermore, people who survive a CVA are at a high risk of recurrence. If the dental team is treating a post-CVA patient or a patient at risk for experiencing a first-time CVA, extreme care must be taken to control anxiety and pain, which could easily trigger a CVA. The CVA presents a difficult emergency for the dental team. It is best to do everything possible to prevent a CVA and to be totally prepared to provide the best treatment possible should one occur.

REVIEW QUESTIONS

MULTIPLE CHOICE

1. A stroke in which signs and symptoms are exhibited for less than a minute is known as a
   a. arteriosclerotic
   b. hemorrhagic CVA.
   c. ischemic CVA.
   d. transient ischemic attack.
2. How many months past a CVA is a patient not a candidate for elective dental care?
   a. 3
   b. 6
   c. 9
   d. 12
3. Which of the following conditions may result in a cerebral hemorrhage?
   a. aneurysm
   b. emboli
   c. thrombosis
   d. ischemia
4. A patient suffering from a stroke should be positioned
   a. in the Trendelenburg position.
   b. in the supine position.

c. upright.
d. in Fowler's position.

5. Which of the following patients have increased chances of experiencing a CVA?
   (1) hypertensive
   (2) diabetic
   (3) history of heart disease
   (4) history of TIA
   a. 1, 2, 3
   b. 2, 3
   c. 1, 4
   d. 1, 2, 3, 4

6. Which of the following are signs or symptoms of a CVA?
   (1)headache
   (2)paralysis
   (3)decreased saliva
   (4)dizziness
   a. 1, 2
   b. 1, 2, 4
   c. 2, 4
   d. 1, 2, 3, 4

7. Which of the following is/are included in the emergency management of a CVA?
   (1)administer a CNS relaxer
   (2)maintain an open airway
   (3)administer oxygen
   (4)summon medical assistance
   a. 1, 2, 3, 4
   b. 1, 2, 4
   c. 2, 3, 4
   d. 1, 3, 4

8. The "A" in the mnemonic "FAST" put forth by The American Red Cross stands for:
   a. Ataxia.
   b. Act.
   c. Arm weakness.
   d. Attack.

9. When scheduling a patient who is at risk for a CVA, what should be considered?
   a. evening appointments are preferable
   b. schedule longer appointments to reduce time the patient needs to return
   c. use maximum amount of epinephrine
   d. use of nitrous oxide sedation to reduce stress

10. Which of the following is not correct regarding documenting medical history for a patient who has a prior history of a CVA?
    a. It is not necessary to document any over-the-counter medications the patient is taking.
    b. Document when the previous CVA occurred.
    c. Document if the patient is compliant with their medications.
    d. Document how long the patient was hospitalized post-CVA.

TRUE OR FALSE

_______ 1. TIAs usually last at least 48 hours.

_______ 2. A thrombus begins when damage occurs to the lining of the blood vessel and the clotting process is initiated.

_______ 3. A cerebral hemorrhage is the most common CVA.

_______ 4. A cerebral thrombosis occurs as a result of an obstruction of the cerebral artery by a clot that forms within the artery.

_______ 5. It is imperative that the dental team know what caused the CVA before it can provide proper management of the CVA.

_______ 6. Paralysis associated with a CVA is usually unilateral.

_______ 7. Signs and symptoms of a CVA can vary according to the area of the brain affected as well as the type of CVA.

_______ 8. People who survive a CVA experience a low risk of recurrence.

_______ 9. Anxiety and pain associated with a dental appointment have the potential to trigger a CVA.

_______ 10. It is uncommon for a patient to experience a TIA prior to experiencing a severe stroke.

MEDICAL EMERGENCY!

CASE STUDY 7-1

A 45-year-old male presents with a positive medical history. He documents on the health history that he is being treated by a physician for hypertension. At the current time his blood pressure is within normal range for his age and gender. While in the office he loses consciousness, then regains consciousness but is unable to speak. The dentist determines that the patient is experiencing a CVA.

Questions

1. State the signs and symptoms of a CVA.

2. Why is the patient's physician's diagnosis an important observation for the dental team to note?

3. State the steps in dental office management of the CVA for this patient.

CASE STUDY 7-2

A 68-year-old female presents with a positive medical history. She states that she has had 6 documented TIAs within the past 12 months. She is in the office for an extraction of a maxillary second molar. She tells you, the dental auxiliary, that she is anxious about the treatment and was unable to sleep the night before due to anxiety. Before the dentist can enter the room, she experiences numbness on one side of her face and body and is having difficulty speaking. You call for the dentist, and as the dentist enters the room, the patient regains feeling on the side that was numb and regains her ability to speak.

Questions

1. Based on her medical history, what might the patient be experiencing?

2. What is this patient at risk for?

3. What is the medical and dental management of this patient?

SECTION THREE

Respiratory Distress Emergencies

This section deals with medical conditions and emergencies that involve the respiratory system.

CHAPTER 8

Asthma

LEARNING OUTCOMES

Upon completion of this chapter, the student will be able to:

- Define asthma
- Compare and contrast the types of asthma
- List the signs and symptoms of asthma
- Describe the treatment provided for an asthma attack
- Discuss the management of an asthmatic attack in the dental office

KEY TERMS

acetylcholine
allergen
bronchioles
cyanosis
extrinsic asthma
intrinsic asthma
sodium hypochlorite
status asthmaticus
stridor
tracheobronchial tree

INTRODUCTION

Diseases or problems associated with the respiratory system such as asthma, bronchitis, or emphysema may create emergency situations. An asthma attack is one example of a respiratory emergency that may occur in the dental setting.

Asthma is a disease of the respiratory tract that can affect all aspects of the **tracheobronchial tree:** trachea, bronchi, and bronchioles (Figure 8-1). It is a chronic lung disorder characterized by constriction of the **bronchioles** (Figure 8-2). There are many different types of asthma, each being brought on by different triggers. The type of a patient is diagnosed with as well as its severity will determine what areas of the tracheobronchial tree are involved. Symptoms vary widely, and ignoring these symptoms can lead to a life-threatening emergency. Asthma affects a large percentage of the population and is not selective as to ethnicity, gender, or age.

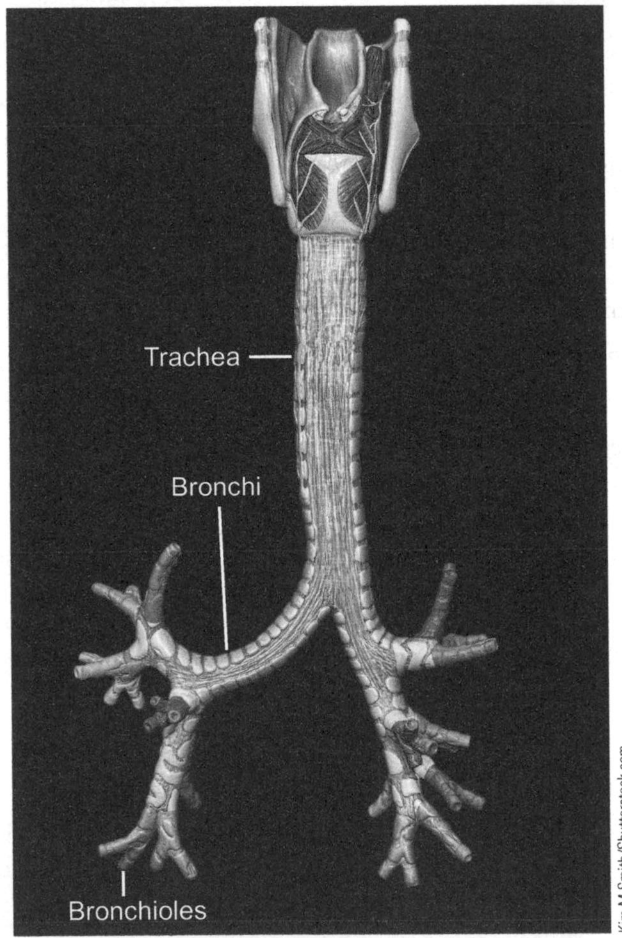

FIGURE 8-1 The tracheobronchial tree consists of the trachea, bronchi, and bronchioles. Asthma affects all aspects of the tracheobronchial tree because it's a respiratory disease.

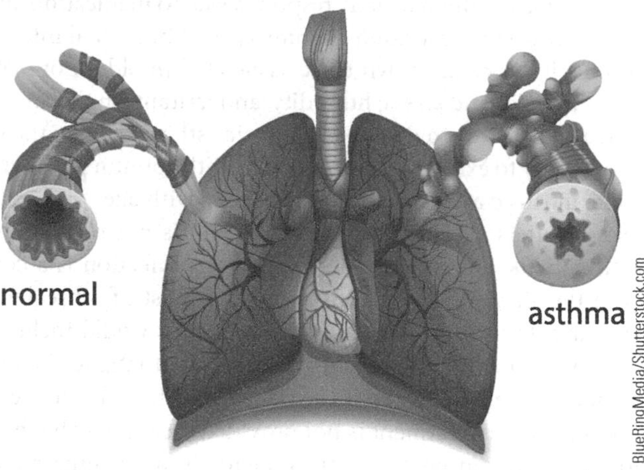

FIGURE 8-2 Normal bronchiole vs. a constricted bronchiole in asthma

TYPES OF ASTHMA

There are two sub-types of asthma, extrinsic and intrinsic. A patient may experience extrinsic or intrinsic asthma independently or may experience a combination of the two.

Extrinsic asthma, or allergic asthma, is a type of asthma that is most commonly diagnosed in children. It makes up the most cases of all asthma conditions, about 60 percent. Episodes of extrinsic asthma usually result from exposure to an **allergen** such as dust, pollen, animals, certain foods, or other substances. Most patients are aware of the types of allergens or conditions that trigger their asthma attacks and try to avoid them. If the allergens are not known, they can be determined by a physician performing allergy tests. In some cases, a person can be allergic to more than one thing. The dental team should also be aware of any specific allergens that trigger a patient's asthma to avoid exposing the patient to them while the patient is in the office. See Emergency Basics 8-1 for a list of common allergens found in a dental office.

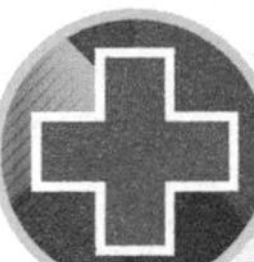

Emergency Basics 8-1

Common Allergens in the Dental Office

- eugenol
- impression materials
- resins
- latex
- local anesthetic agents (very rare)
- amalgam
- **sodium hypochlorite**

The extrinsic asthmatic patient usually does not exhibit any signs or symptoms of asthma between episodes. Furthermore, extrinsic asthma usually responds well to medication and *may* be outgrown.

Intrinsic asthma usually occurs as a result of some type of bronchial infection. It has also been called nonallergic asthma. It has been shown to be associated in older populations. Some triggers could include infections, exercise and stress, humidity, and irritants in the air. A doctor would need to have bloodwork and a chest X-ray to diagnose intrinsic asthma. Unlike the extrinsic asthma patient, this patient is more likely to exhibit a chronic cough with sputum production between attacks. Unlike extrinsic asthma, intrinsic asthma usually progresses with age.

In the event a person suffers a severe asthma attack and is not responding to treatment, this can lead to **status asthmaticus**. Often, an upper respiratory infection is a common cause due to the mucous buildup in the airway. This is considered the most life-threatening type of asthma. If someone is experiencing status asthmaticus, their symptoms would include diminished breath sounds, **cyanosis**, sweating, shortness of breath, wheezing, and fatigue. The patient experiencing status asthmaticus is not responding to the medications that have been prescribed and must be treated in a hospital. If immediate treatment is not provided, death may be the result.

Anxiety or emotional upset can be a triggering factor in an asthma attack in someone who has a history of asthma. It is also one of the main causes of asthma attacks in the dental office. For example, some anxious children can experience an asthma attack immediately on entering the dental operatory. It is extremely important for the dental staff to do everything possible to prevent emotional upsets by using stress reduction protocol as outlined in Table 5-3. Some highly anxious patients may benefit from sedation with nitrous oxide or an oral medication such as Valium prior to dental treatment. Sedation would reduce the risk of an asthmatic attack.

A patient with mild asthma that may be managed with inhalers is an ASA II. A patient with moderate to severe asthma may be an ASA III. Patients who have been hospitalized previously for asthma are also an ASA III.

TEST YOUR KNOWLEDGE

1. What type of asthma is considered the most life-threatening?

2. What type of asthma is usually reported in young children?

3. What type of asthma usually occurs as a result of a bronchial infection?

4. What are some allergens that are found within a dental operatory?

5. What are some of the symptoms of status asthmaticus?

SIGNS AND SYMPTOMS

An asthma attack may occur suddenly without any warning or slowly over an extended period. The first step when dealing with an asthmatic patient in an emergency is to distinguish between asthma and an airway obstruction. If there is confusion, listen to the sounds the patient is making. With airway obstruction, **stridor**—a constant-pitch musical sound—may be heard during inhalations. With asthma, a wheezing sound heard during expirations is characteristic. In addition, an easy way to determine that the patient is suffering from an asthma attack is to also be aware of the patient's health history. If the patient exhibiting signs and symptoms has indicated a history of asthma, the attack should be treated as asthma.

During an asthma attack, the bronchioles become narrowed due to contractions of the smooth muscles, and there is an overproduction of mucus. As a result, the air passages are restricted, breathing becomes difficult, and the patient seems to be struggling for air. With asthma, exhaling is the most difficult part of breathing, although most of the time the patient feels as if inhaling is the most difficult part.

The patient suffering from an asthma attack may be sweating and coughing and may appear to be very nervous. The nervousness occurs as a result of the patient's inability to breathe normally. The patient may also complain of a severe tightness in the chest. It is also common for blood pressure and pulse to increase slightly during an attack. However, in some cases, these vital signs may remain close to the baseline readings.

The duration of an asthma attack varies from patient to patient. If left untreated, the attack may continue anywhere from a few minutes to several hours. The patient usually experiences a severe coughing attack and expectorates a large bolus of mucus just before the attack terminates. If the patient is treated immediately with a bronchodilator, the attack usually ends within a few seconds. Some patients with severe asthma may be prescribed steroid medications to manage their disease. Steroid medications are not meant to treat an acute asthmatic attack. Steroids help to reduce bronchiole inflammation and minimize the risk and severity of an asthma attack. Steroid medications may be inhaled or may be oral. Status asthmaticus, as already noted, is the most severe form of asthma. It may begin like any other asthma attack but will not respond to any type of treatment or medication, and the patient therefore experiences one continuous asthma attack. In some cases, status asthmatic occurs because the patient was not compliant with prescribed steroid medication. The situation may continue for days. This person is in a life-threatening situation and should be hospitalized immediately.

See Emergency Basics 8-2 for signs and symptoms of asthma.

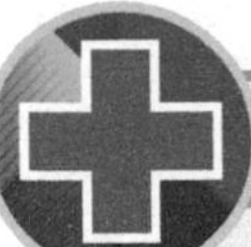

Emergency Basics 8-2

Asthma Signs and Symptoms

- Coughing
- Sweating
- Tightness in chest
- Difficulty breathing
- Wheezing
- Blood pressure normal or elevated
- Increased heart rate
- Nervousness

TEST YOUR KNOWLEDGE

1. What is the sound heard if the patient is experiencing an asthma attack?
2. If treated with a bronchodilator, how long does an asthma attack last?

TREATMENT OF ASTHMA

Once it has been determined that a patient is suffering from an asthma attack, prompt management should be administered as follows:

1. Stop all dental treatment. Be sure to remove all materials and instruments from the patient's mouth. The patient will be breathing forcibly, so make sure there are no cotton rolls or other small items left in the mouth for the patient to inhale.
2. Position the patient. Raise the patient upright; since the patient will be struggling for air, the patient will be more comfortable if seated upright.
3. Use a bronchodilator. The bronchodilator is an aerosol medication that relaxes the bronchioles and makes it easier for the patient to breathe (Figure 8-3). The health history will state whether the patient suffers from asthma. Once this information is established, the dental auxiliary should ask the patient whether they are carrying a bronchodilator prior to the start of the treatment session (Figure 8-4a). If so, the patient's bronchodilator should be placed within easy

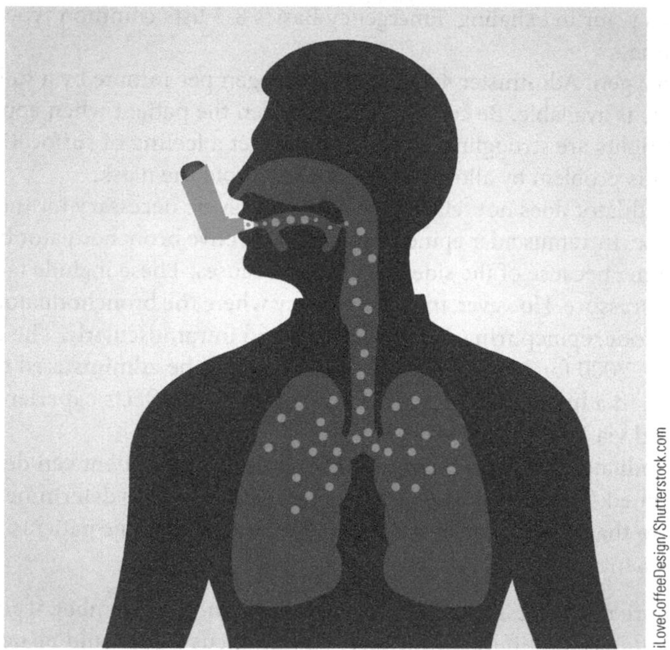

FIGURE 8-3 Epinephrine in the bronchodilator relaxes the bronchioles during an asthma attack.

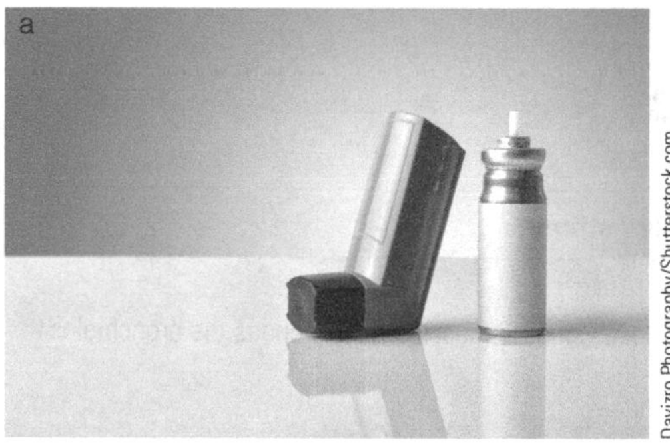

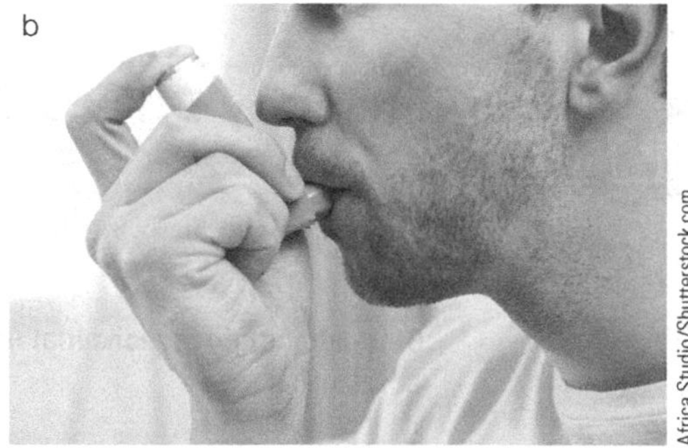

FIGURE 8-4 (a) Inhaler with bronchodilator medication cartridge; (b) patient administering an inhaler during an asthma attack.

reach in case an attack occurs. If an attack does take place, allow the patient to self-administer the bronchodilator; patients know what their usual dose involves (Figure 8-4b). In the event the patient does not have their own bronchodilator, the one from the emergency kit should be retrieved and administered to the patient. The patient will insert the bronchodilator in their mouth and breathe in slowly as they depress the inhaler each time. The patient will hold their breath for 10 seconds prior to exhaling. Emergency Basics 8-3 lists common types of bronchodilators used for asthma.

4. Administer oxygen. Administer 4 to 6 liters of oxygen per minute by a full-face mask or nasal cannula, if one is available. Be careful not to frighten the patient when applying the face mask. Asthmatic patients are struggling for air and may get a feeling of suffocation from the oxygen mask. Solve this problem by allowing the patient to hold the mask.
5. If the bronchodilator does not relieve the attack, it may be necessary for the dentist to administer epinephrine. Intramuscular epinephrine is an effective bronchodilator but is not the drug of choice in asthma because of the side effects that it causes. These include tachycardia and elevation of blood pressure. However, in an emergency where the bronchodilator is not resolving the asthmatic episode, epinephrine can be administered intramuscularly. The doses are 1:1,000 for an adult and 1:2,000 for a child. These doses should not be administered through an IV as the epinephrine is in a highly concentrated form and the side effects experienced would be severe if administered via IV.
6. If the bronchodilator alleviates the attack, the clinician and patient can determine if treatment may be continued. The patient may prefer to reschedule. Always determine what led to the asthmatic attack so that triggers can be avoided at the next visit. Some patients may opt for sedation prior to treatment.

If these steps are not successful, call for medical assistance. Remember, if all treatment is unsuccessful, the patient may be suffering from status asthmaticus and should be hospitalized as soon as possible.

See Emergency Basics 8-4 for a summary of the management of an asthmatic attack in the dental office.

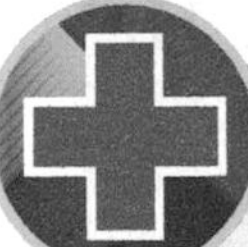

Emergency Basics 8-3

Common Bronchodilator medicines for asthma

1. **Beta-adrenergic bronchodilators**–relaxes smooth muscles, which opens the bronchioles
   a. albuterol
   b. levalbuterol
   c. epinephrine injection
2. **Anticholinergic bronchodilators**–blocks the effect of **acetylcholine**, which stimulates muscles and constricts the airway
   a. ipratropium
   b. tiotropium
3. **Xanthine derivatives**–suppresses response for airway to stimuli, relaxes the smooth muscle.
   a. theophylline
   b. aminophylline

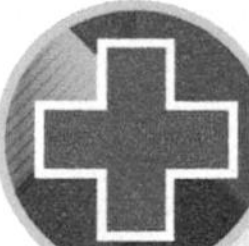

Emergency Basics 8-4

Management of an Asthma Attack in the Dental Office

1. Stop dental treatment.
2. Position patient upright.
3. Administer bronchodilator.
4. Administer oxygen.
5. Administer epinephrine if the bronchodilator is not alleviating the asthmatic attack and summon medical help.

TEST YOUR KNOWLEDGE

1. Where should the patient's bronchodilator be placed during treatment?

2. How should a patient be positioned after it has been determined that the patient is experiencing an asthmatic episode?

SUMMARY

Asthma attacks in the dental office are most often triggered by anxiety. Therefore, it is extremely important to try to keep all patients calm, especially the asthmatic patient. If an asthma attack does occur, try to reassure the patient while administering prompt, efficient treatment and management.

REVIEW QUESTIONS

MULTIPLE CHOICE

1. Which of the following is not a sign or symptom of asthma?
   a. wheezing
   b. tightness in the chest

c. coughing
d. stridor

2. What is administered by the patient to relieve asthma during an attack?
   a. injection
   b. bronchodilator
   c. IV
   d. tablet

3. What type of asthma is considered the most life-threatening?
   a. status asthmaticus
   b. intrinsic asthma
   c. extrinsic asthma
   d. infectious asthma

4. An example of a beta-adrenergic bronchodilator is:
   a. albuterol.
   b. theophylline.
   c. aminophylline.
   d. ipratropium.

5. What type of asthma is usually reported in young children?
   a. extrinsic
   b. infectious
   c. intrinsic
   d. none of the above

6. Which of the following is not a part of management for a patient suffering from an asthma attack in the dental office?
   a. administer oxygen.
   b. place patient in supine position.
   c. administer bronchodilator.
   d. administer epinephrine.

7. Which of the following is not a sign or symptom of asthma?
   a. coughing
   b. tightness of chest
   c. wheezing
   d. low blood pressure

8. Extrinsic asthma is more common in children. Intrinsic asthma is more common in adults.
   a. Both statements are true.
   b. Both statements are false.
   c. The first statement is true. The second statement is false.
   d. The first statement is false. The second statement is true.

9. Stridor is a commonly heard sound during an asthmatic attack. Stridor is usually heard during inhalation.
   a. Both statements are true.
   b. Both statements are false.
   c. The first statement is true. The second statement is false.
   d. The first statement is false. The second statement is true.

10. Intrinsic asthma is triggered by an allergen. Extrinsic asthma is usually triggered by an infection.
   a. Both statements are true.
   b. Both statements are false.
   c. The first statement is true. The second statement is false.
   d. The first statement is false. The second statement is true.

TRUE OR FALSE

_______ 1. An asthma attack may occur suddenly or can be ongoing for a long period of time.

_______ 2. Oxygen should not be administered to the asthmatic patient.

_______ 3. A patient suffering from status asthmaticus should be hospitalized as soon as possible.

_______ 4. Asthma only begins in young children.

_______ 5. If epinephrine is necessary, the dentist would administer intramuscular 1:1,000 for an adult and intramuscular 1:2,000 for a child.

_______ 6. Asthma is a disease that is characterized by constriction of the bronchioles.

_______ 7. Those with intrinsic asthma usually outgrow it.

_______ 8. Steroid medications may be used to treat an acute asthmatic attack.

_______ 9. Epinephrine is the drug of choice in an asthmatic attack.

_______ 10. It is important to implement a stress reduction protocol in a patient with a history of asthma.

MEDICAL EMERGENCY!

CASE STUDY 8-1

A 55-year-old female presents in the dental office for a crown preparation with final impressions on tooth number 30. As the auxiliary seats the patient, she asks the patient if there have been any changes in her medical history. The patient states that her physician has given her a bronchodilator. The procedure concludes with no complications and the dentist leaves the treatment room. As the patient is preparing to leave, she begins to cough, and the auxiliary observes that the patient is having difficulty breathing. The auxiliary looks for the patient's bronchodilator.

Questions

1. What type of asthma attack is the patient most likely experiencing?
2. What should the auxiliary have done prior to the beginning of treatment?
3. What other condition could the patient be experiencing?

CASE STUDY 8-2

A 10-year-old male presents to the dental office with a positive history of extrinsic asthma. The patient is there today to have two teeth extracted for orthodontic purposes. The dentist is running behind and the patient has to wait for 20 minutes before he is taken into the operatory. Once seated, the patient begins to cough, wheeze, and struggle to breathe. The dentist, aware of the patient's medical history, sends the auxiliary to the waiting room to retrieve the bronchodilator from his mother. During this time, the dentist speaks calmly to the patient. The bronchodilator is administered, and the patient recovers completely.

1. How could keeping the patient in the waiting room increase the chances of an asthmatic attack occurring?
2. Where should the patient's bronchodilator have been prior to treatment?
3. What was the main trigger of the patient's asthmatic attack?

CHAPTER 9

Hyperventilation

LEARNING OUTCOMES

Upon completion of this chapter, the student will be able to:

- Define hyperventilation
- Explain the causes of hyperventilation
- Describe the best way to prevent hyperventilation
- Explain the physiology of hyperventilation
- Describe the signs and symptoms of hyperventilation
- Discuss the management of hyperventilation

KEY TERMS

alkalosis	diazepam	myocardial infarction
carbon dioxide	hypocarbia	perioral

INTRODUCTION

Hyperventilation is an increase in the rate or depth of breathing that results in a change in the blood chemistry. It usually occurs as a result of anxiety and/or panic. The dental office can be an anxious setting for most people, which is why hyperventilation is a one of the more common emergencies that may occur.

CAUSES OF HYPERVENTILATION

In addition to being caused by anxiety, hyperventilation also may be caused by certain physical conditions, emotional upset, or stress. These other causes are usually not the cause of an episode of hyperventilation in the dental office.

Hyperventilation is not normally encountered in children. Children usually cry or scream when frightened, which expresses their fears and prevents hyperventilation from occurring. This is because children exhibit their fears and usually do not internalize them. Hyperventilation occurs most often in patients age 15 to 45 years who hide their feelings and do not admit their fears of dentistry. In such patients, the anxiety builds up within until they can no longer control it. Children usually cry or scream when frightened, which expresses their fears and prevents hyperventilation from occurring.

PREVENTION OF HYPERVENTILATION

Identification of the anxious patient is important in the prevention of an episode. Refer to Chapter 2 to review the anxiety questionnaire, which helps aid in identifying the anxious patient. The patient may also be asked about previous unpleasant experiences in the dental office.

Use vital signs as well for aid in identification. The apprehensive patient may have an elevated blood pressure and pulse rate. It is critical to obtain baseline vitals when the patient is not anxious, preferably at the initial visit.

PHYSIOLOGY OF HYPERVENTILATION

Hyperventilation is characterized by tachypnea. By increasing respirations, the person exhales a large amount of **carbon dioxide** (CO_2) and there is an excess of oxygen (O_2) in the blood in relation to CO_2. The result is **hypocarbia** and respiratory **alkalosis**, which must be reversed to restore a normal oxygen and carbon dioxide balance.

For instance, in comparison to an athlete who has performed strenuous exercise, there is an increase in the depth and rate of respirations. However, in the athlete, the exercised muscles release carbon dioxide into the blood, which replenishes the excess CO_2 given off by the rapid breathing. Because dental patients are motionless, they have no way of replenishing the carbon dioxide being exhaled. As a result, patients can suffer from a lack of carbon dioxide and have difficulty breathing.

Hyperventilation takes place in a cycle. First, the patient becomes very anxious about the dental treatment. This results in the patient beginning to hyperventilate. Next, the patient begins to realize they are having difficulty breathing. This then makes the patient more anxious, which worsens the hyperventilation (Figure 9-1). This cycle will increase in severity unless someone intervenes. The patient may feel a tightness

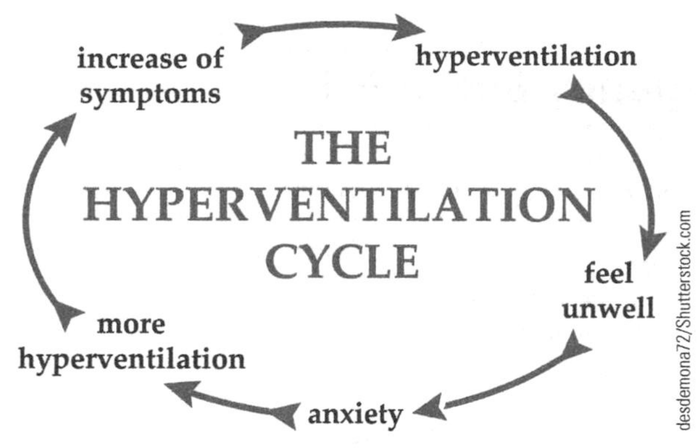

FIGURE 9-1 The hyperventilation cycle

TEST YOUR KNOWLEDGE

1. Which group of patients is most unlikely to experience hyperventilation?
2. The patient who hyperventilates is experiencing a lack of what gas?
3. What is the most common cause of hyperventilation in the dental office?

in their chest and feel as if they are having a **myocardial infarction.** It is of utmost importance for members of the dental team to recognize the problem, intervene, and attempt to calm the patient.

SIGNS AND SYMPTOMS OF HYPERVENTILATION

A patient first entering the operatory may appear nervous or anxious but usually does not discuss any fear of the dental procedure. At the onset of hyperventilation, the patient begins to breathe deeper and faster. At this point, the patient usually does not realize there has been a change in their breathing pattern. The patient may then complain of a feeling of suffocation and tightness in the chest. As the patient continues to hyperventilate, they may experience a feeling of dizziness. If the episode is allowed to continue, tingling may develop in the extremities and the **perioral** areas. Patients experiencing hyperventilation are in respiratory distress, although they will not be cyanotic as in other cases (e.g., an airway obstruction) because they are receiving plenty of oxygen.

See Emergency Basics 9-1 for a summary of the signs and symptoms of hyperventilation.

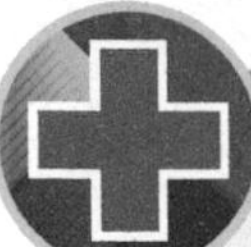

Emergency Basics 9-1

Signs and Symptoms of Hyperventilation

- Nervousness
- Increase in rate of respirations
- Feeling of suffocation
- Tightness in chest
- Dizziness
- Tingling in extremities and perioral areas

TEST YOUR KNOWLEDGE

1. What are the signs and symptoms of hyperventilation?
2. How do the rate and depth of respiration affect the hyperventilating patient?

MANAGEMENT OF HYPERVENTILATION

Hyperventilation is an emergency situation that usually can be corrected by performing the following steps:

- The patient will need to be calmed in order for them to cooperate.
- The patient can then be asked to cup their hands and cover their nose and mouth. Encourage the patient to breathe the exhaled, carbon dioxide–rich air slowly as this will reverse the hypocarbia (Figure 9-2).
- If this is not successful, Valium may need to be administered to the patient; in this case, the patient will need to be driven home by a family member. Valium is not a first choice in management of hyperventilation and should be used as a last resort if the dental professional is not able to calm the patient so they can cooperate.

Emergency Basics 9-2 provides the steps necessary for management of an episode of hyperventilation.

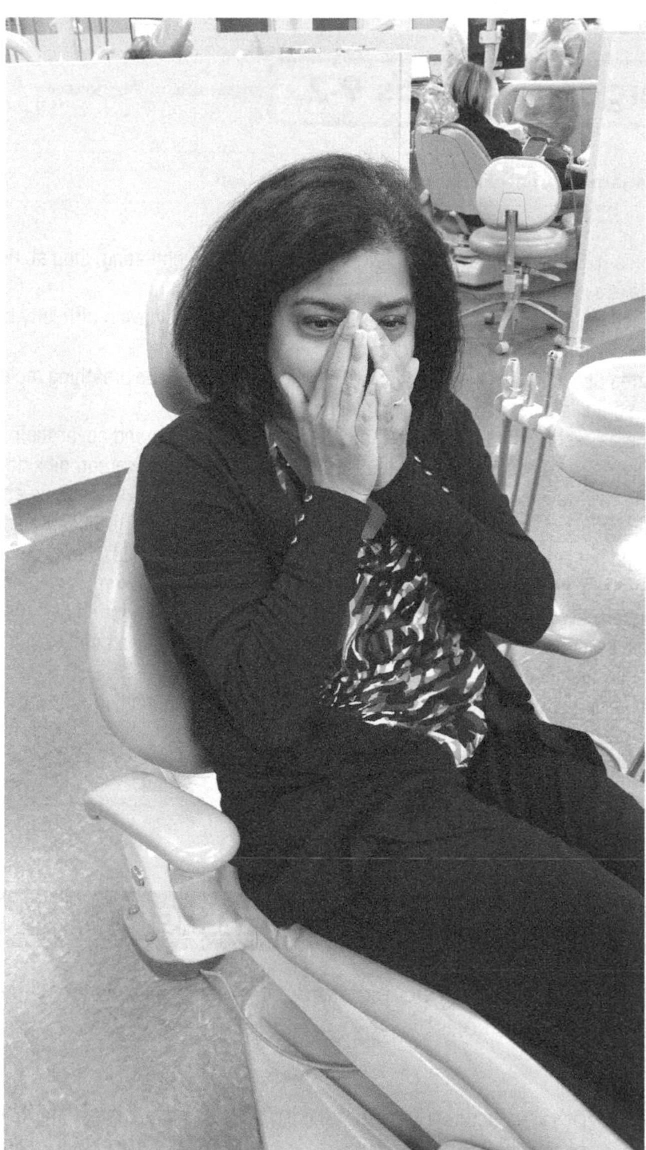

FIGURE 9-2 A patient who is hyperventilating cups their hands over their nose and mouth and rebreathes carbon dioxide–rich air into the body

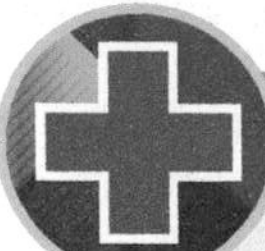

Emergency Basics 9-2

Management of an Episode of Hyperventilation

1. Once it has been determined that the patient is hyperventilating, stop all dental treatment. Make sure to remove any objects from the patient's mouth.
2. Place the patient in an upright position. A patient who is having difficulty breathing will be more comfortable sitting upright.
3. Attempt to calm the patient, who will be agitated and will be breathing rapidly. Speak to the patient in a quiet and reassuring manner.
4. The easiest method is to have the patient cup their hands and cover their nose and mouth (Figure 9-1). Encourage the patient to breathe the exhaled, carbon dioxide–rich air slowly. This will reverse the hypocarbia. Never administer oxygen to a hyperventilating patient. Remember, this patient already has too much oxygen and too little carbon dioxide.
5. If the patient is experiencing a severe hyperventilation episode, it may be necessary for the dentist to administer a drug to reduce anxiety. **Diazepam** (Valium) is a commonly prescribed antianxiety drug. If this step is necessary, prepare the prescription and the patient instruction according to the dentist's guidelines. The patient will then need to be sent home with a family member.
6. Determine what caused the episode so that treatment modifications can be made for the next appointment. The patient may need sedation for the next visit if they are anxious about dental care.

TEST YOUR KNOWLEDGE

1. What is usually the drug administered if medication is used to treat the hyperventilating patient?
2. Why is a hyperventilating patient instructed to breathe into their hands cupped over their nose and mouth?
3. What should never be administered to a patient who is hyperventilating?

SUMMARY

Hyperventilation in the dental office usually occurs as a result of anxiety and/or panic. After an episode, it is important for the dental team to determine what caused the patient's fears of dentistry. Once this has been established, it will be easier for the team to take steps to alleviate the fears and, it is hoped, to prevent another hyperventilation episode.

REVIEW QUESTIONS

MULTIPLE CHOICE

1. Which of the following groups is most likely to experience hyperventilation?
   a. young adults
   b. young children
   c. elderly
   d. all the above
2. The patient who hyperventilates is suffering from a lack of which of the following?
   a. carbon dioxide
   b. oxygen
   c. nitrogen
   d. hydrogen
3. Which of the following is a common cause of hyperventilation?
   a. overexertion
   b. being happy
   c. being relaxed
   d. anxiety
4. Which of the following is a sign or symptom of hyperventilation?
   a. nervousness
   b. tacyhpnea
   c. feeling of suffocation
   d. all the above
5. What is usually the drug administered if medication is required to calm the patient to reverse hyperventilation?
   a. diazepam
   b. Dilantin
   c. epinephrine
   d. oxygen

6. Anxiety can lead to an episode of hyperventilation in the dental office. Children are most likely to exhibit hyperventilation when anxious.
   a. Both statements are true.
   b. Both statements are false.
   c. The first statement is true, the second statement is false.
   d. The first statement is false, the second statement is true.

7. A hyperventilating patient may feel as if they are having a myocardial infarction. This is caused by a feeling of tightness in their chest.
   a. Both statements are true.
   b. Both statements are false.
   c. The first statement is true, the second statement is false.
   d. The first statement is false, the second statement is true.

8. The patient who is hyperventilating may feel tingling in which of the following areas?
   a. hands
   b. feet
   c. perioral
   d. all of the above

9. Identification of an anxious patient is important in preventing an episode of hyperventilation in the dental office. The anxiety questionnaire is a good tool to use to identify an anxious patient.
   a. Both statements are true.
   b. Both statements are false.
   c. The first statement is true, the second statement is false.
   d. The first statement is false, the second statement is true.

10. Which of the following Is correct regarding management of a hyperventilating patient?
    a. The patient should be placed in the supine position.
    b. The patient should immediately be given Valium to calm them down.
    c. The patient should be asked to breathe into a paper bag.
    d. The operator should speak calmly to the patient to reassure them.

TRUE OR FALSE

______ 1. Hyperventilation is one of the most uncommon emergencies experienced in the dental office.

______ 2. Hyperventilation usually can be relieved by having the patient breathe into a plastic bag.

_______ 3. The rate and depth of respirations increase dramatically in the hyperventilating patient.

_______ 4. Hyperventilation usually results in a lack of oxygen.

_______ 5. The hyperventilating dental patient should be placed in the supine position.

_______ 6. Valium is the drug of choice for management of hyperventilation.

_______ 7. Hyperventilation leads to hypercarbia.

_______ 8. Hyperventilation leads to respiratory alkalosis.

_______ 9. Oxygen should be administered to the hyperventilating patient.

_______ 10. The patient who is hyperventilating has an excess of oxygen.

MEDICAL EMERGENCY!

CASE STUDY 9-1

A 35-year-old female patient presents with a negative medical history. She has come to the office to have an amalgam placed in tooth number 20. Once seated in the dental chair, the patient begins to talk rapidly and clutches the arms of the chair. She admits no fear of the dental procedure but appears to be very nervous and then begins to breathe rapidly and complains of tightness in the chest and a feeling of suffocation. She is hyperventilating.

Questions

1. Describe the management protocol for this patient.

2. How could the dental auxiliary prevent this situation from occurring on the patient's next visit?

3. Why should oxygen not be administered in this situation?

CASE STUDY 9-2

A 25-year-old female presents for routine dental treatment. This appointment is her second visit. On the first visit, she was very anxious but tolerated the procedures well. At this appointment, the patient is kept waiting in the operatory for a longer period due to the duration of another patient's treatment. As the dentist prepares to administer the local anesthesia, the auxiliary notes that the patient is beginning to breathe rapidly and deeply.

Questions

1. What condition is the patient most likely experiencing?

2. What is the management for this condition?

3. What could the auxiliary have done to prevent this episode?

CHAPTER 10

Airway Obstruction

LEARNING OUTCOMES

Upon completion of this chapter, the student will be able to:

- Explain possible causes of airway obstruction in the dental office
- Discuss methods to prevent airway obstruction in the dental office
- Describe the anatomy of the airway
- Compare and contrast the various types of airway obstructions
- Choose the appropriate management for the various types of airway obstructions
- Define the Heimlich maneuver
- Discuss the rationale for a cricothyrotomy

KEY TERMS

asphyxiation	cricothyrotomy	Heimlich maneuver	tracheotomy
aspirate	dental dam	trachea	

INTRODUCTION

Every aspect of the human body depends on the availability of adequate oxygen to function properly. Depriving the body of oxygen for even a few minutes can lead to irreversible brain damage and ultimately to death. It is therefore of utmost importance to recognize and manage an airway obstruction both quickly and correctly. Airway obstruction is not selective; young and old alike can be victims.

CAUSES OF AIRWAY OBSTRUCTION IN A DENTAL OFFICE

An airway obstruction may occur in a dental office setting. The development of sit-down dentistry, which places the patient in the supine position, has increased the incidence of dental patients **aspirating** objects into the airway. Practically every aspect of dentistry requires that some object be placed into or taken out of the patient's oral cavity. These objects, when coated with saliva or blood, can easily slip out of the dentist's or auxiliary's hands and cause an obstruction in the patient. Some items that may be aspirated and produce obstructions as well as how aspiration can be prevented are listed in Emergency Basics 10-1.

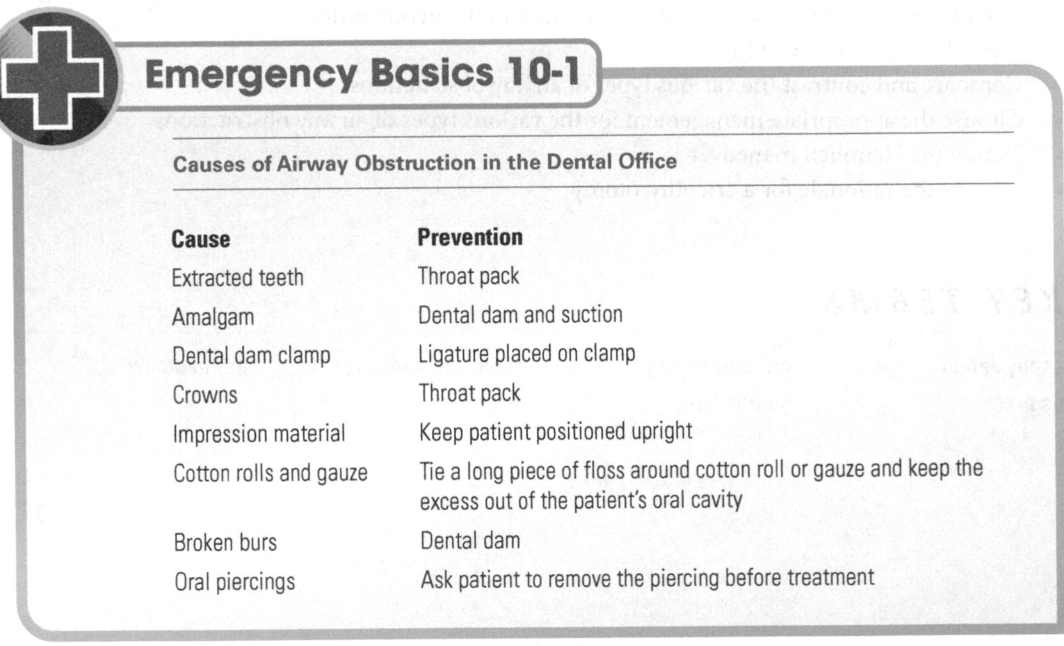

Emergency Basics 10-1

Causes of Airway Obstruction in the Dental Office

Cause	Prevention
Extracted teeth	Throat pack
Amalgam	Dental dam and suction
Dental dam clamp	Ligature placed on clamp
Crowns	Throat pack
Impression material	Keep patient positioned upright
Cotton rolls and gauze	Tie a long piece of floss around cotton roll or gauze and keep the excess out of the patient's oral cavity
Broken burs	Dental dam
Oral piercings	Ask patient to remove the piercing before treatment

The use of certain protective devices such as the **dental dam** (Figure 10-1) helps prevent a number of possible airway obstructions. However, some methods of treatment make it impossible to use this

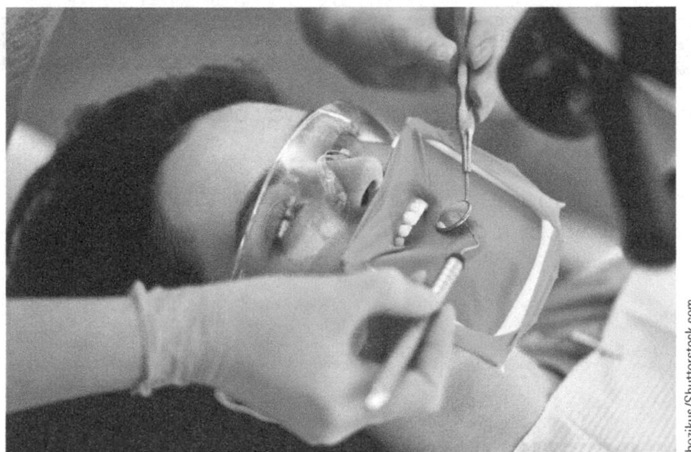
bezikus/Shutterstock.com

FIGURE 10-1 Dental dam

device; in these cases, extra precautions must be taken. The auxiliary should be assertive with the high-volume evacuator and have the cotton pliers available to retrieve any dropped object.

If an object is dropped, it is extremely important to remain calm to keep the patient from overreacting. Most of the time the patient's gag reflex will allow the patient to cough the object back into the oral cavity where it can be removed. It is important to note, if the patient is sedated, their protective gag reflex may not be fully functional, and the risk of aspiration increases.

Oral Piercing

Body piercing has become a more prevalent form of body art in today's society. Oral piercing, which may involve the tongue, lips, uvula, or a combination of sites, has been implicated in several adverse oral conditions, including:

- Gingival injury or recession
- Damage to teeth or restorations
- Interference with speech or chewing and swallowing
- Scar tissue formation
- Prolonged bleeding
- Severe infection

An emergency related to oral piercing may present in the form of an airway obstruction. The jewelry can become dislodged and move into the airway. When dental personnel are providing treatment for a patient with some form of oral piercing, they should take precautions to avoid dislodging the jewelry.

Because of the potential for various related complications, the American Dental Association opposes the practice of oral piercing. Some dental offices will ask the patient to remove their oral piercings for their dental appointment, if possible, to prevent any emergency situations.

TEST YOUR KNOWLEDGE

1. What are some common causes of airway obstruction in the dental office?

2. When making an impression on a patient, what is the best way to prevent an airway obstruction?

ANATOMY OF THE AIRWAY

Most airway obstructions that dental personnel will encounter occur in the upper airway. To know what occurs during an obstruction, it is important to understand the anatomy of the upper airway. Figure 10-2 is an illustrated view of upper airway anatomy. The mouth and nose empty into a

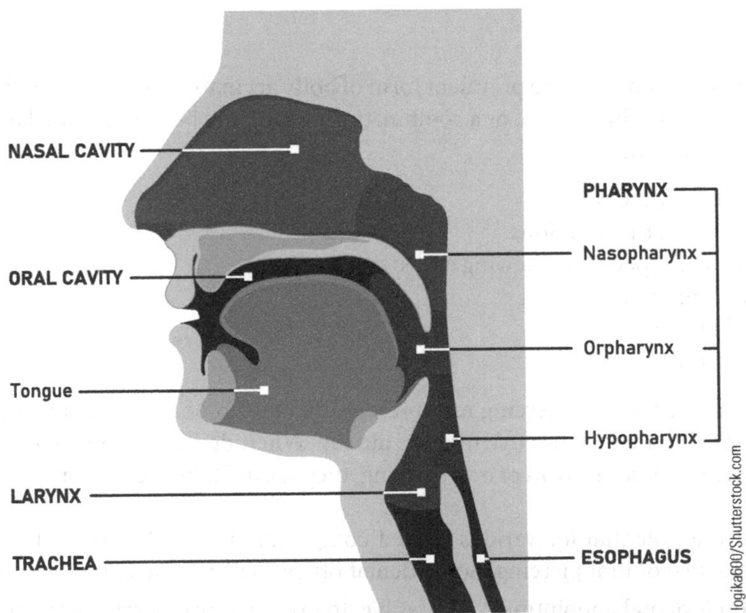

FIGURE 10-2 Structures of the upper respiratory tract

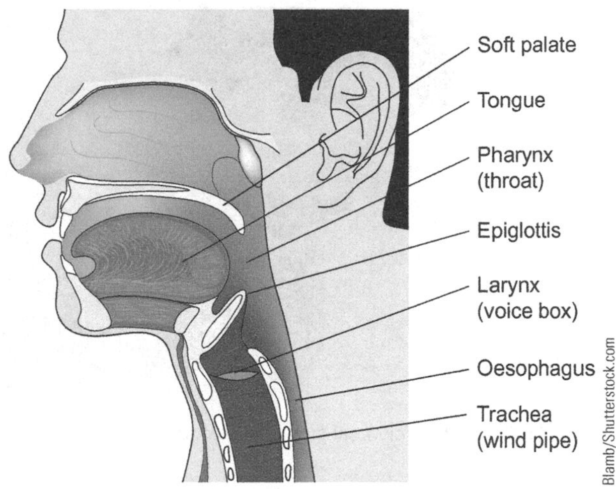

FIGURE 10-3 Epiglottis closes to prevent swallowed food from entering trachea

common passage called the pharynx, or throat. The pharynx is further broken up by location. The upper part of the pharynx behind the nose is the nasopharynx. The middle is the oropharynx, and the lower part is the hypopharynx. The hypopharynx ends where the next two passages begin. The first passage is the **trachea.** The trachea, also commonly called the windpipe, is the largest passage, located in the front of the throat, and carries air from the pharynx into the lungs. The second passage is the esophagus, located behind the trachea, which carries solids and liquids from the mouth to the stomach.

When food is swallowed, it is kept out of the trachea by the epiglottis, a flap that covers the opening of the trachea whenever food approaches (see Figure 10-3). In some cases, food or other objects get past the epiglottis and pass into the trachea. The majority of the time the patient coughs and the object is removed. However, in some instances the object becomes lodged in the trachea, and an airway obstruction occurs. The upper-airway anatomy is completed by the larynx, or voice box. (The lower airway consists of the bronchi, alveoli, and lungs.)

TYPES OF AIRWAY OBSTRUCTIONS

Airway obstructions can result from a number of situations such as trauma, foreign objects, secretions, burns, or tumors. No matter what the cause, several different types of airway obstructions may occur. The different degrees of airway obstruction require different techniques to treat them. See Emergency Basics 10-2.

A *partial airway obstruction* occurs when the airway is not completely blocked. In this situation some air gets through to the lungs. A partial obstruction can be one with adequate air exchange or one with inadequate air exchange. A patient experiencing a partial obstruction with adequate air exchange will cough forcibly. This person is able to talk and may try to explain that the object

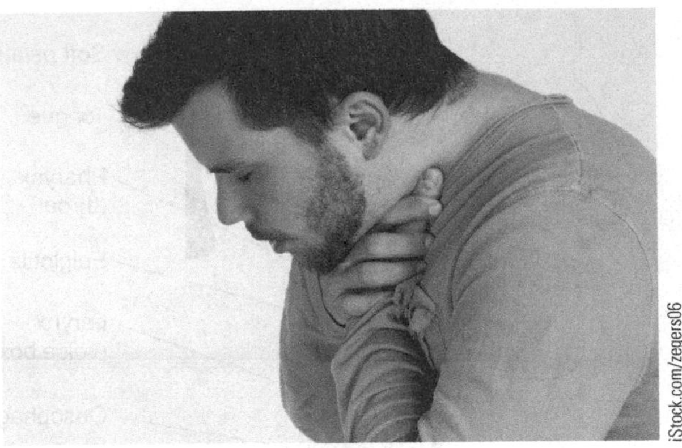

iStock.com/zegers06

FIGURE 10-4 Universal sign for choking

"went down the wrong way." Such a person is usually not in serious trouble and should be encouraged to cough.

The patient experiencing a *partial obstruction with inadequate air exchange* is certainly in danger. This person will not cough, although a crowing sound will be made that is a result of the air passing over the lodged object. As the episode progresses, the person may show signs of cyanosis around the mouth because of the lack of oxygen. The main problem with this situation is that it can easily become a complete airway obstruction. This patient may not be receiving enough oxygen to sustain life and may lose consciousness, suffer brain damage, or die.

The *complete airway obstruction* is the most life threatening. The individual suffering from this condition is not able to make any noise but may exhibit the universal distress signal, clutching the throat with the hands (Figure 10-4). The person usually panics immediately and may resist treatment. A person suffering from a complete airway obstruction becomes extremely pale and **cyanotic** and may die from **asphyxiation** in approximately four to six minutes, risking irreversible brain damage and eventually death. It is of utmost importance that this condition be diagnosed and treated immediately.

TEST YOUR KNOWLEDGE

1. In which type of airway obstruction can the patient talk and explain the condition?

2. Which type of airway obstruction is the most life threatening?

THE HEIMLICH MANEUVER

Throughout history people have had various remedies for choking; in most cases the treatments were unsuccessful. Dr. Henry Heimlich developed a technique for relieving airway obstructions that has become known as the **Heimlich maneuver** and consists of a series of manual abdominal thrusts. The Heimlich maneuver makes use of the air that remains in the victim's lungs. The pressure placed on the abdomen during manual thrusts causes an elevation of the diaphragm, which increases pressure on the lungs and causes an explosive force of air to be released and hopefully to clear the trachea. Chest thrusts, and not abdominal thrusts, should be used on a pregnant patient who is experiencing airway obstruction. Since the invention of the Heimlich maneuver, there has been a great deal of controversy over its use. Injuries such as fractured ribs have resulted from the maneuver being performed incorrectly. However, the Heimlich maneuver has been found to be successful unless the object cannot be removed, the maneuver is done incorrectly, or too much time elapsed before the technique was started. The dental auxiliary should be trained in BLS/CPR, which includes the Heimlich maneuver technique. It is important to complete regular refresher courses to maintain a current BLS/CPR certification.

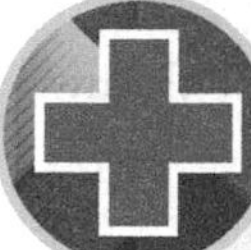

Emergency Basics 10-2

Treatment of Airway Obstructions

Partial Obstruction with Adequate Air Exchange	Encourage patient to cough. Most of the time, the object is expelled.
Partial Obstruction with Inadequate Air Exchange	Patient may not be receiving adequate oxygen. This patient should be treated as if suffering from a complete airway obstruction. Heimlich maneuver should be performed.
Complete Airway Obstruction	Perform the Heimlich maneuver.

TEST YOUR KNOWLEDGE

1. What is the Heimlich maneuver?

2. What is the treatment for a patient with a partial airway obstruction with adequate air exchange?

CRICOTHYROTOMY

No matter how well the Heimlich maneuver is performed, in some situations it may not be successful. If such a situation arises, it may be necessary to use surgical intervention. Any type of surgical airway intervention, however, should only be done by someone who is trained and qualified in its use, and only as a last resort.

Formerly, the method of choice was a **tracheostomy.** However, the area where it must be performed is close to several large sources of blood and nerve supplies. Therefore, this technique can easily cause severe problems even when performed in the best of circumstances. It requires more expertise and is intended for a more long-term maintenance of the airway. As a result, the **cricothyrotomy** has replaced the tracheotomy as the treatment of choice when an emergency airway must be provided. A cricothyrotomy is performed as follows:

Locate the cricothyroid ligament (or cricothyroid membrane) by placing the finger on the Adam's apple and sliding downward toward until you feel a slight indented area. This is the cricothyroid ligament. (See Figure 10-5.)

1. Using a sharp object, preferably a scalpel, make an incision in this area, and then widen the incision. There will be little bleeding because there are no major blood vessels in this area.
2. The opening must be maintained. Place an item such as a suction tip or your finger into the incision to keep the airway open. If necessary, artificial respiration may be administered through this temporary air space.

A modification of this technique is use of the cricothyrotomy needle. Practically every emergency kit contains such an item. The needle has a very large diameter, usually 14 gauge, which permits air to pass through. The method detailed above is used with one exception: instead of making an incision, the needle is inserted into the cricothyroid membrane. (See Figure 10-6.)

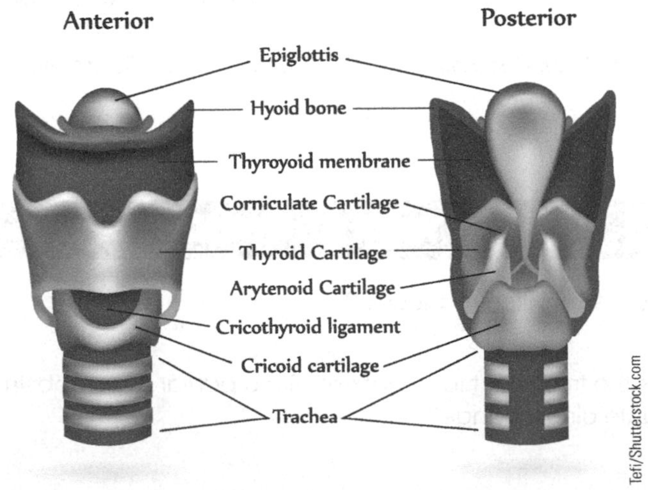

FIGURE 10-5 Cricothyroid ligament location

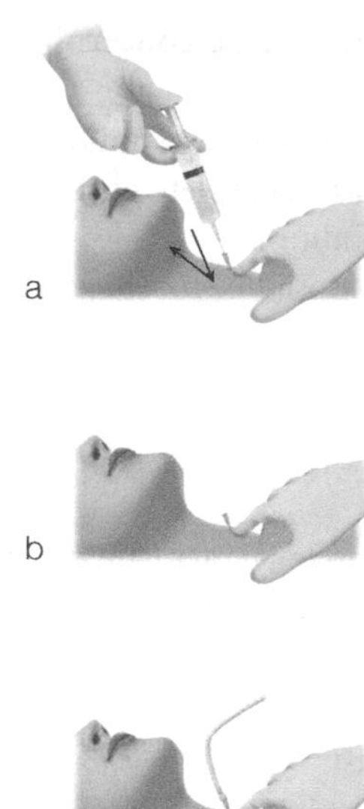

FIGURE 10-6 a) Insert a saline filled syringe at a 30° to 40° angle into the cricothyroid ligament; b) Once hub is even with the skin, remove needle' and c) Attach an oxygen supply

Source: From Roberts and Hedges' Clinical Procedures in Emergency Medicine, 6th ed, 2013

SUMMARY

An airway obstruction can occur at any time to any patient. Brain damage or death can occur very quickly as a result of an airway obstruction. It is therefore of utmost importance that the dental auxiliary quickly recognize and effectively treat the condition.

REVIEW QUESTIONS

MULTIPLE CHOICE

1. What is the trachea commonly known as?
   a. voice box
   b. throat
   c. windpipe
   d. none of the above

2. Which of the following is true concerning a partial obstruction with inadequate air exchange?
   (1) patient may exhibit a crowing sound
   (2) should be treated as a complete obstruction
   (3) is not a serious condition
   (4) patient may be cyanotic
   a. 1, 2, 3, 4
   b. 1, 2, 3
   c. 2, 3, 4
   d. 1, 2, 4

3. What should be the management be for a patient suffering from a partial obstruction with adequate air exchange?
   a. encourage coughing
   b. use the full Heimlich
   c. use manual thrusts only
   d. all of the above

4. Which patient would benefit most from chest thrusts if experiencing an airway obstruction?
   a. pregnant patient
   b. tall patient
   c. unconscious patient
   d. all the above

5. What is the universal distress signal to indicate an airway obstruction?
   a. placing the palm of the hand over the mouth
   b. clutching the throat with both hands
   c. covering the eyes with the palms of both hands
   d. none of the above

6. What is the most accepted surgical technique for relieving an airway obstruction?
   a. cricothyrotomy
   b. tracheotomy
   c. laryngectomy
   d. none of the above

7. Sit-down dentistry with the patient in the supine position has led to a decrease in object aspiration. Objects become slippery with blood or saliva, increasing the risk of aspiration.
   a. Both statements are true.
   b. Both statements are false.
   c. The first statement is true, the second statement is false.
   d. The first statement is false, the second statement is true.

8. Which of the following methods is the best way to prevent aspiration of dental amalgam?
   a. dental dam
   b. throat pack
   c. use of ligature
   d. keep patient upright

9. Oral piercings do not pose a risk for airway obstruction. However, oral piercings can damage teeth or existing restorations.
   a. Both statements are true.
   b. Both statements are false.
   c. The first statement is true, the second statement is false.
   d. The first statement is false, the second statement is true.

10. Which of the following is not correct regarding the pharynx?
    a. The nasopharynx is located behind the nose.
    b. The middle part of the pharynx is the oropharynx.
    c. The lower part of the airway is the hypopharynx.
    d. The mouth and nose empty into the hypopharynx.

TRUE OR FALSE

________ 1. Brain damage can occur as a result of a lack of oxygen in as little as four to six minutes.

________ 2. The use of the rubber dam may help prevent some airway obstructions.

________ 3. The Heimlich maneuver is usually not successful.

________ 4. Most airway obstructions experienced by dental health care workers occur in the upper airway,

________ 5. Chest thrusts are best performed on pregnant patients.

________ 6. The epiglottis covers the opening of the esophagus when food approaches.

________ 7. It is not possible for an airway obstruction to occur in the dental office setting.

________ 8. A tracheotomy is the procedure of choice in the event an airway obstruction cannot be cleared through other methods.

________ 9. A person with a complete airway obstruction may exhibit cyanosis.

________ 10. Aspiration of extracted teeth can be prevented with the use of a throat pack.

MEDICAL EMERGENCY!

CASE STUDY 10-1

A 16-year-old male presents in the dental office with a negative medical history. He has come to the dental office to have a crown cemented on number 30. During the try-in the crown slips from the dentist's hand and enters the patient's throat. The patient begins to gasp and make a crowing sound. The dental team gets the patient out of the chair and begins to perform the Heimlich. After two sequences, the object is expelled and the patient recovers.

Questions

1. What type of obstruction is the patient experiencing?

2. What could have been done to prevent this situation from occurring?

CASE STUDY 10-2

A 32-year-old female presents in the dental office with a positive medical history. She is in her second trimester and is six months pregnant. The patient is scheduled to have impressions made for a whitening tray. The dental auxiliary places the patient in a supine position and inserts the upper impression tray. The patient begins choking and experiencing airway obstruction with inadequate air exchange.

Questions

1. How could this emergency have been prevented?

2. What modifications of the Heimlich maneuver should be performed with this patient?

SECTION FOUR

Cardiovascular Emergencies

This section deals with medical conditions and emergencies that involve the cardio-vascular system.

CHAPTER 11

Angina Pectoris and Myocardial Infarction

LEARNING OUTCOMES

Upon completion of this chapter, the student will be able to:

- Name the major parts of the heart
- Explain how atherosclerosis affects the coronary arteries
- Describe the progression of coronary artery disease
- Define angina pectoris
- Differentiate between stable and unstable angina
- List three precipitating factors of angina
- Describe the signs and symptoms of angina
- Explain how the dentist may recognize angina
- List two side effects of nitroglycerin
- Describe the steps in the management of an angina attack
- Discuss dental management of the patient with a history of angina
- Define myocardial infarction
- Describe the signs and symptoms of myocardial infarction
- Describe the management for myocardial infarction
- Compare and contrast angina and myocardial infarction
- Explain what the dental team can do to prevent angina or myocardial infarction from occurring in the dental office

KEY TERMS

amyl nitrite
angina pectoris
anticoagulant
antihypertensive
aorta
arteriosclerosis
atria
atrioventricular valves

congestive heart failure
coronary artery disease
diuretic
endocardium
epicardium
epigastrium
hypoxia
ischemia
lumen
myocardial infarction
myocardium
orthostatic hypotension
pericardium
pulmonary artery
semilunar valves
substernal
ventricles
warfarin

According to the Centers for Disease Control, cardiovascular disease is the leading cause of death in the United States today. Heart disease may present itself in several ways, but this chapter is limited to two types of heart disease that may present emergency situations in the dental office: angina pectoris and acute myocardial infarction.

ANATOMY OF THE HEART

To understand how certain diseases or conditions affect the heart, it is important to understand some of the basic anatomy of the heart.

Several structures combine to make up the four-chambered, hollow, muscular organ known as the heart. The **pericardium** is the wall, or sac, that encloses the heart. This wall is made up of three layers: the external layer, called the **epicardium**; the middle layer, called the **myocardium**; and the inner layer, called the **endocardium** (see Figure 11-1). Each layer has special characteristics or responsibilities. First, coronary vessels must pass through the epicardium before entering the myocardium. Second, the myocardium consists of muscle fibers that give the heart the ability to contract. Third, the endocardium lines the cavities of the heart, covers the valves, and, to some extent, lines the large blood vessels.

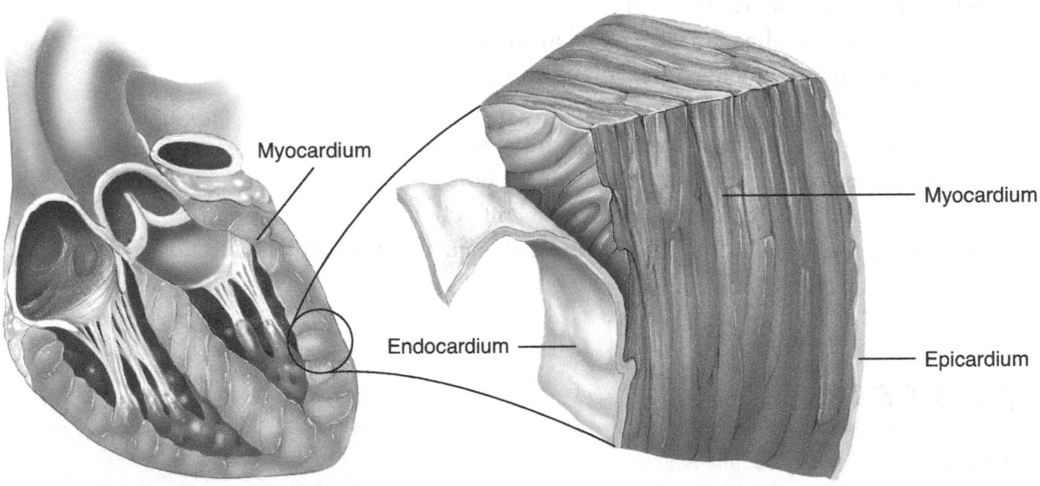

FIGURE 11-1 Types of tissues that make up the heart muscle: myocardium, epicardium and endocardium.

The heart consists of four chambers. The upper chambers are called the **atria** and are separated into right and left sides by the interatrial septum. The lower chambers are called the **ventricles** and are divided into right and left sides by the interventricular septum. Refer to Figure 11-2 for anatomy of the human heart.

The right atrium receives deoxygenated blood from all tissues except the lungs. This blood is then pumped to the right ventricle, from which the **pulmonary artery** exits and carries blood to the lungs. The left atrium receives oxygenated blood from the lungs by way of the pulmonary veins. Oxygenated blood then enters the left ventricle, which is connected to the **aorta**. The aorta pumps oxygenated blood to all parts of the body except the lungs.

Contained within the heart's chambers are two kinds of valves: the **atrioventricular valves** and the **semilunar valves**. The atrioventricular valves consist of the tricuspid and mitral valves, and the semilunar valves consist of the pulmonary and aortic valves (refer to Figure 11-2). The atrioventricular valves separate the atria from the ventricles. The right atrium and ventricle are separated by the tricuspid valve, and the left atrium and ventricle are separated by the mitral valve. The valves allow blood to be pumped from the atria to the ventricles when the atria contract and then prevent blood from re-entering the atria when the ventricles contract.

The semilunar valves work similarly, although their location is different. The pulmonary valve is located between the right ventricle and the pulmonary artery, and the aortic valve is located between the left ventricle and the aorta.

The heart is best known as the organ that provides blood to the rest of the body, but, to survive, the heart muscle itself must receive an adequate supply of oxygenated blood. The myocardium is supplied with blood by the first branches of the aorta, the right and left coronary

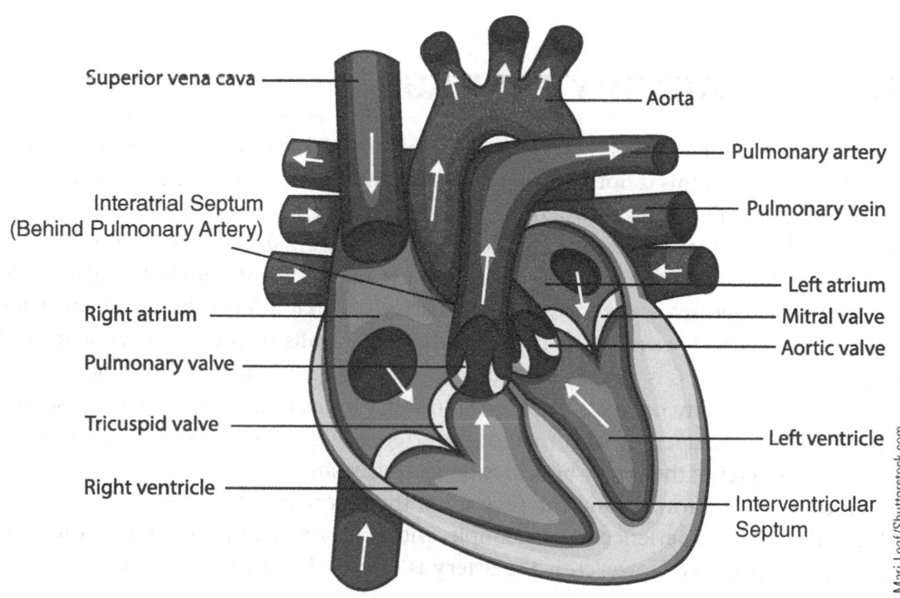

FIGURE 11-2 Anatomy of the human heart

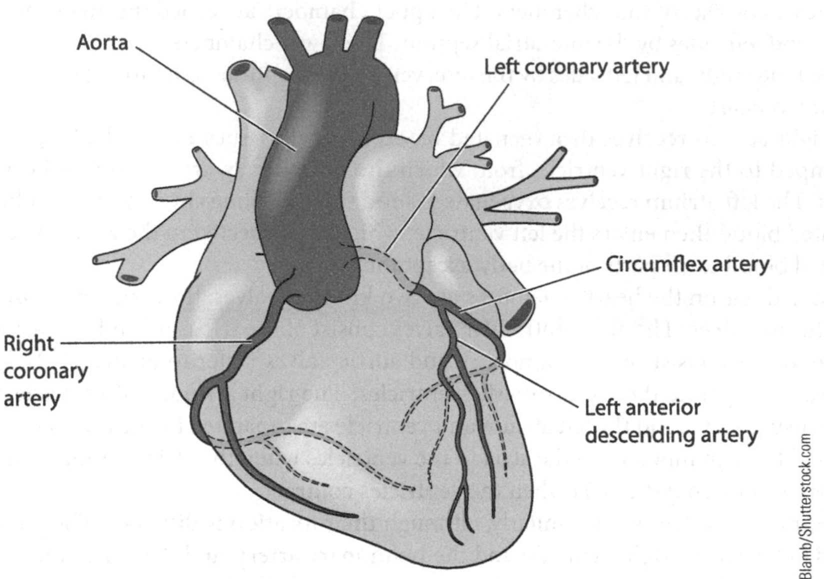

FIGURE 11-3 Coronary arteries of the heart

arteries (Figure 11-3). The left main coronary artery supplies blood to the left ventricle and left atrium. The right main coronary artery supplies blood to the right ventricle and the right atrium.

CORONARY ARTERY DISEASE

Both physical and emotional stress can cause the heart to work harder and therefore require more oxygen. In a healthy heart this is not a problem, because the vessels dilate and the heart receives more oxygenated blood on call. However, when the heart is diseased, this dilation does not take place.

A common disease that causes this problem is **arteriosclerosis**, more commonly called hardening of the arteries, in which the artery walls become thickened and inelastic (also discussed in Chapter 7). Atherosclerosis is the form of arteriosclerosis that affects the coronary arteries and causes **coronary artery disease**. With this condition, the walls of the coronary arteries become thick and hard. The process is usually gradual and may take years to develop. The process begins with small amounts of fatty deposits or plaques in the arteries that with time increase in size and cause a narrowing of the opening or **lumen** of the arteries (Figure 11-4). Calcification follows, and eventually the diameter of the artery becomes dangerously small.

The degree of this narrowing and the severity of the coronary artery disease determine the adverse effects the patient experiences. For example, with a narrowing of the arteries, the patient may experience angina pectoris. However, if the artery is extremely narrow or perhaps even occluded,

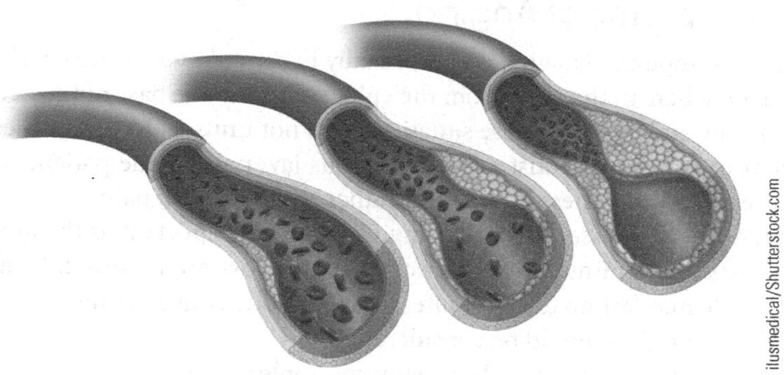

FIGURE 11-4 Stages of Arteriosclerosis: (a) beginning cholesterol build-up, (b) advanced cholesterol build-up, and (c) complete blockage

myocardial infarction may occur. Coronary artery disease can progress over time. A patient may experience angina for a period of time and then, as the disease increases in severity, experience a myocardial infarction.

TEST YOUR KNOWLEDGE

1. What layer of the heart enables the heart to contract?

2. What is the difference between arteriosclerosis and atherosclerosis?

3. How does the progression of fatty deposits affect the disease process?

ANGINA PECTORIS

Angina pectoris is a Latin phrase that means a "strangling of the chest." Angina is characterized by episodes of pain when the heart experiences oxygen deficiency. This oxygen deficiency may be caused by conditions that result in decreased blood flow to the heart, decreased capacity of the blood to carry oxygen, or increased workload in the heart. A diminishment of the oxygen supply to the heart muscle results in myocardial **ischemia** or **hypoxia**. In some cases, angina is the first sign of atherosclerotic disease of the coronary arteries.

Signs and Symptoms of Angina

The most common symptom of angina is pain, usually in the **substernal** area of the chest, although it can be located anywhere in the chest from the **epigastrium** to the base of the neck. The pain may also spread to the jaw and teeth. In these situations, it is not unusual for even an edentulous (without teeth) patient to consult a dentist with continuous jaw pain. Some patients may describe the condition as a pressure or tightness in the chest rather than as actual pain.

The duration of the pain associated with angina is just as important as the location. An angina episode usually lasts 3 to 5 minutes if the precipitating factors are removed. If the factors are not removed, the episode may last up to 40 minutes. If the episode continues much longer, the possibility of a myocardial infarction should be considered.

During an episode, the patient usually remains motionless in an attempt to alleviate the pain. In most cases the pain ceases within minutes, and the patient may continue activity. However, if the patient does not stop activity at least for a short period, the pain worsens until it becomes almost unbearable. On the other hand, in a few patients the pain may stop without cessation of the physical activity. This recovery can be possible because the collateral channels may start to function, which decreases myocardial hypoxia. The increase in the oxygen levels that are occurring with alternate pathways will help to reduce the patient's discomfort and pain.

The physical signs in an angina attack usually are not reliable. Appearance may remain relatively normal, or the patient's skin may appear pale or gray in color and become cold and clammy. The pulse rate and blood pressure may increase slightly before or coincidentally with the onset of an angina attack. The increase in pulse rate and blood pressure is the central nervous system's way of trying to increase the oxygen flow to the myocardium. The patient may also experience a feeling of impending doom. Emergency Basics 11-1 summarizes the list of common signs and symptoms of an angina attack.

TEST YOUR KNOWLEDGE

1. What is the appearance of someone experiencing an angina attack?

2. What is a common first sign of atherosclerotic disease of the coronary arteries?

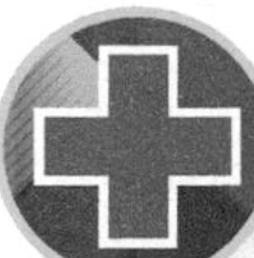

Emergency Basics 11-1

Signs and Symptoms of Angina

- Substernal chest pain
- Patient remains motionless
- Normal appearance or paleness/grayness
- Cold, clammy skin
- Increase in pulse rate
- Increase in blood pressure
- Feeling of impending doom

Classifications of Angina

Angina pectoris is most often classified as either stable or unstable. Pain from stable angina usually occurs as a result of physical exertion or emotional upset. Stable angina usually does not alter in frequency, duration, or intensity within a 60-day period, whereas unstable angina changes. Unstable angina is unpredictable in regard to cause, with episodes occurring even at rest. Attacks often increase in frequency, severity, and duration. Attacks that were once controlled by nitroglycerin may require a higher dosage or become completely immune to its effects. See Emergency Basics 11-2 for a comparison of stable and unstable angina.

The amount of stress necessary to cause an attack can vary from time to time, and an angina episode may occur at any time of day or night. See Emergency Basics 11-3 for a list of possible precipitating factors of angina episodes.

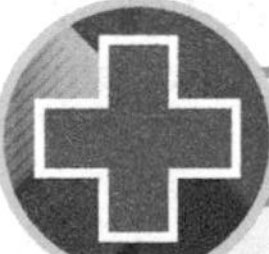

Emergency Basics 11-2

Comparison of Stable and Unstable Angina

Stable Angina
- Pain results from physical or emotional stress
- No alteration in duration, frequency, or intensity
- Controlled with nitroglycerin

Unstable Angina
- Pain may occur even at rest
- Often increases in duration, frequency, or intensity
- May require increase in dosage of nitroglycerin, or nitroglycerin may have no effect

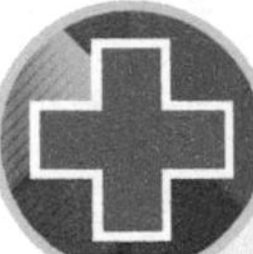

Emergency Basics 11-3

Precipitating Factors of Angina Episodes

- Physical exertion
- Emotional stress
- Eating or drinking cold foods
- Dressing
- Bathing
- Sexual activity
- Disturbing dreams
- Eating a heavy meal

Recognition of Angina

If the patient experiences chest pain while in the dental office, the dentist must attempt to determine the cause. The first course of action is to recheck the patient's medical history for any notations of angina or other cardiac problems. If the health history does not identify any history of heart disease, the patient should be asked some specific questions:

1. *What type of discomfort are you experiencing?* It is best not to ask what type of pain the patient is experiencing because some people may not describe the condition as pain. Rather, they may describe the condition as being like a clamping down on the chest or like someone is standing on the chest. Others may describe the condition as an ache or a dull, burning sensation. If the patient describes a sharp or knifelike pain, the condition is probably not angina pectoris.
2. *Describe the location of your discomfort.* Angina pectoris pain is not usually well localized. If the patient can point to one small area where the pain is occurring, the problem is most likely not angina. Most often angina is felt in the substernal area in the middle of the chest. The pain may radiate down either or both arms and may cause a feeling of numbness. The pain may also radiate to the neck or jaw.
3. *Have you had this type of discomfort in the past, and if so, how long did your discomfort last?* Angina pain is usually steady, with little change in intensity, and may last from a minute to several hours. However, the longer the pain lasts, the greater the chances of the patient experiencing a myocardial infarction. Pain that fluctuates or lasts only a few seconds is usually not angina.
4. *What preceded the discomfort in the past?* Angina pain is usually brought on by physical exertion or emotional stress. Exposure to cold weather or eating a large meal may also be a precipitating factor. It is beneficial for the dental team to be aware of the precipitating factors to prevent a recurrence of the attack.
5. *What provided relief from your discomfort in the past?* If relief comes after resting for a few minutes, taking nitroglycerin, or both, the condition is most likely angina. Remember, however, that this is a tricky situation, since some other serious heart conditions may mimic these symptoms.

Since the basic symptoms of most heart conditions are similar, the emergency diagnosis may depend on the patient's response to certain treatment. For example, if the patient is treated with nitroglycerin and the pain is not relieved, the condition may be myocardial infarction rather than angina.

TEST YOUR KNOWLEDGE

1. What are characteristics of unstable angina pectoris?

2. What are precipitating factors of angina pectoris?

3. What is the most common symptom of angina pectoris?

Management of an Angina Attack

Management of angina is multifaceted through the use of nitroglycerine as well as rest. Both are discussed in this section. The dental auxiliary plays an important role in keeping the patient calm and assisting the dentist with managing the emergency. The dental assistant may be asked to retrieve the emergency kit and to summon emergency medical services (EMS).

Nitroglycerin Nitroglycerin is a coronary vasodilator prescribed for the prevention or relief of angina. Its function is to help dilate the coronary arteries to allow more oxygenated blood to reach the heart. Sublingual nitroglycerin has become the accepted drug for the relief of angina episodes because of its rapid action. Nitroglycerin that is administered sublingually will dissolve and can be rapidly absorbed through the highly vascularized mucosa under the tongue. On average, effects of nitroglycerin are noticeable within 90 seconds after sublingual administration of the correct dose.

Nitroglycerin also can be administered in pill form, as a spray, or through a transdermal patch. The transdermal patch is placed on clean dry skin once a day and is commonly used in the prophylactic treatment of angina (see Figure 11-5). Some patients may use a topical ointment form of nitroglycerin, which they place on the chest before participating in a physical activity they feel may trigger an attack.

Individual sensitivity to nitroglycerin varies, so a physician will determine the correct dose for each individual. For this reason, it is important to allow patients to administer their own nitroglycerin if possible.

Two common side effects are associated with the use of nitroglycerin. First, **orthostatic hypotension** can occur (it may be corrected with dose adjustments). Second, severe headaches may result when nitroglycerin administration is first started. Most clinicians have observed the disappearance

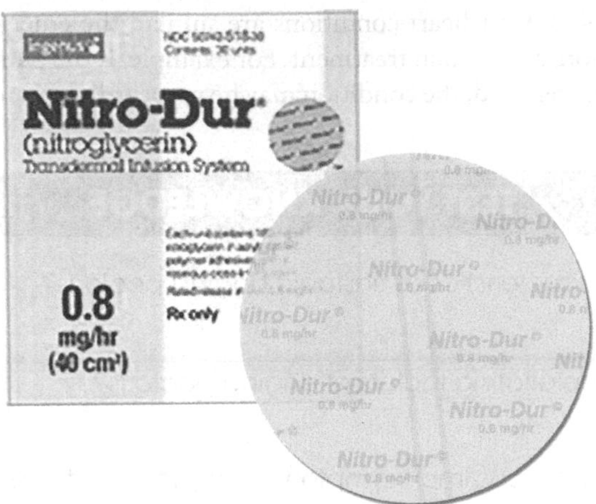

FIGURE 11-5 Transdermal nitroglycerin patch Nitro-Dur® is one way to manage angina pectoris

Source: National Institutes of Health (NIH)

of these initial headaches during the continued administration of the nitroglycerin. Additionally, nitroglycerine causes facial flushing due to the ability to dilate blood vessels.

Nitroglycerin starts to work rapidly and should improve the patient's condition within approximately 90 seconds after it is administered. If it is not effective, the nitroglycerin may be expired, which is why nitroglycerin should be stored in its original bottle with the cap tightly sealed. Nitroglycerine tables last for 3 to 6 months after the bottle has been opened. Sublingual nitroglycerine causes a tingling sensation when administered. If the patient does not experience this, the medication is expired and the sublingual spray from the emergency kit should be retrieved and administered. Nitroglycerine may not be effective if the atherosclerosis is so severe that the drug is no longer effective and other medication may be needed or if the patient may be experiencing a myocardial infarction. Although nitroglycerin alone allows most angina sufferers to lead normal lives, in some cases additional drugs, such as beta blockers, may also be required.

Management Steps for an Angina Attack Once the dentist has determined the patient's condition as angina pectoris, the goal of treatment must be to reduce the demand of the heart muscle for oxygen. This is achieved by the following:

1. *Remain calm.* It is vital that the patient have confidence in the ability of the dental team to manage the situation, especially if this is the first time the patient has experienced an angina attack. The dental team should alleviate as much anxiety as possible.
2. *Stop all dental treatment.* Make sure to remove all items from the patient's mouth. Also make sure to remove from the patient's sight all items that may have been causing concern or anxiety, such as syringes.
3. *Position the patient upright* as that will usually be most comfortable.
4. *Administer nitroglycerin.* Ask patients who have reported a medical history of angina if they have their nitroglycerin with them, and if they do, place the medication within easy reach at the beginning of the appointment. Patients who have a history of angina know the duration and intensity of the pain. Most emergency kits contain nitroglycerin, but it is best that patients

administer their own, since the dosage has been determined to meet their needs. When administered, the nitroglycerin should be placed sublingually and allowed to dissolve. If the patient does not have a positive medical history for angina, the chest pain should be managed as a myocardial infarction and 911 should be called immediately; management of a myocardial infarction will be discussed later in this chapter. If a patient tells you that the pain is different from their usual angina pain, they may be experiencing a myocardial infarction. If the patient does have a history of angina and does not have their own nitroglycerin, proceed to administer the nitroglycerin available in the emergency kit.

5. *Administer oxygen.* Since the patient is suffering from a lack of oxygenated blood reaching the heart, administering oxygen makes the patient more comfortable.
6. *If the angina is not relieved* by the first dose of nitroglycerin, a second dose may be administered after 5 minutes. Up to three doses may be administered within a 15-minute time period.
7. *If the management described is unsuccessful* in relieving the patient's symptoms, the dental team should assume the patient is experiencing myocardial infarction rather than angina and treat accordingly.

Note: If nitroglycerin is not available, **amyl nitrite** may be administered. However, in some instances unpleasant side effects have been associated with this drug, so administer it only if nitroglycerin is not available. Side effects of amyl nitrite can include spontaneous voiding of the bladder, loss of sphincter control of the large intestine, nausea, vomiting, syncope, hypotension, and an abnormally fast heart rate.

MANAGEMENT OF THE DENTAL PATIENT WITH A HISTORY OF ANGINA

The patient experiencing angina, especially the first time, will be frightened and upset. Most associate the chest discomfort with impending death, primarily because most people know someone who has died from a heart problem. This concern increases the need for oxygen going to the heart and therefore has a tendency to worsen the condition. The dental team must work to relieve the fear brought about by this association. This may be accomplished by prompt treatment to relieve the chest discomfort, maintaining control of the situation, and reassuring the patient.

It is always better to prevent an angina attack from occurring in the dental office than to have to manage an episode, because an angina attack can lead to myocardial infarction and even to cardiac arrest and death. Prevention is accomplished through proper management of the patient with a history of angina and by being aware of the patient's medical history as well as taking steps to alleviate stress from the dental visit. Stress reduction protocol is beneficial in preventing an angina attack. Sedation with nitrous oxide and oxygen will allow the patient to be more relaxed and aid in the prevention of an angina attack. Excellent pain control with 2 cartridges of lidocaine 1:100,000 will be beneficial to the patient as well. Additionally, the patient may take their nitroglycerine as a preventive prior to the start of the appointment. Table 11-1 provides medical history items that are specific to heart disease. Table 11-2 provides predisposing factors for angina.

TABLE 11-1 Medical History and Prevention of an Acute Angina Attack

- Patients who had a myocardial infarction or a cerebrovascular accident in the past could be on aspirin therapy and may also be taking potent **anticoagulants** such as **warfarin** to prevent a recurring incident.
- Question the patient about previous heart disease or a family history of heart disease.
- Diabetics and those with adrenal and thyroid disorders are at a significantly higher risk for cardiovascular disease than those without these disorders.
- Those with a positive history of angina should be questioned regarding the frequency and duration of episodes as well as the factors that trigger an angina attack. Record details about the radiation of the pain during an attack and how well nitroglycerine alleviates an attack.
- For those with a history of angina, request that the patient bring nitroglycerine to each appointment; be sure to check the expiration date of the medication. At each appointment, the patient's nitroglycerine should be kept within reach in the event of an angina episode during dental treatment.

TABLE 11-2 Predisposing Factors for Angina

- Diabetics are more prone to developing cardiovascular problems and as a result angina.
- High blood pressure, if left untreated, leads to cardiovascular damage and angina.
- Hypertension can cause angina.
- Obesity is usually caused by poor diet and a sedentary lifestyle.
- Family history of cardiovascular disease increases the risk of angina.
- Elevated cholesterol levels are linked to angina.
- Males over the age of 45 are prone to cardiovascular disease.
- Smokers are more likely to develop cardiovascular disease, leading to angina.

With all dental patients, it is important to try to ensure a visit that is pain-free, but this is especially important with patients who have a history of coronary problems. Pain tends to cause stress, which will aggravate a heart condition and possibly trigger an attack. It may be necessary to limit the length of dental appointments for patients with a heart condition, since the stress placed on such patients by long appointments may trigger an emergency.

TEST YOUR KNOWLEDGE

1. What is the most common medication used to treat angina pectoris?

2. What effect does it have on the coronary arteries that makes it the drug of choice for a patient having an angina attack?

3. What is the management of a patient who is experiencing an angina attack?

MYOCARDIAL INFARCTION

When there is a significant narrowing or a blockage of the coronary arteries, a condition known as **myocardial infarction** may occur. Myocardial infarction is included in the section with angina because in some cases angina attacks may advance to myocardial infarction. On the other hand, myocardial infarction may occur in a patient who has never experienced an angina episode.

Myocardial infarction is a condition that occurs when a portion of the myocardium dies as a result of oxygen starvation caused by the narrowing or complete blockage of the artery that supplies that area with blood (refer to Figure 11 6 for a detailed illustration). The condition may be created by any problem that causes an inadequate supply of oxygenated blood to reach the myocardium, a common cause being atherosclerosis.

TEST YOUR KNOWLEDGE

1. What is occurring to the heart muscle during a myocardial infarction?

2. Why is the heart muscle experiencing this event?

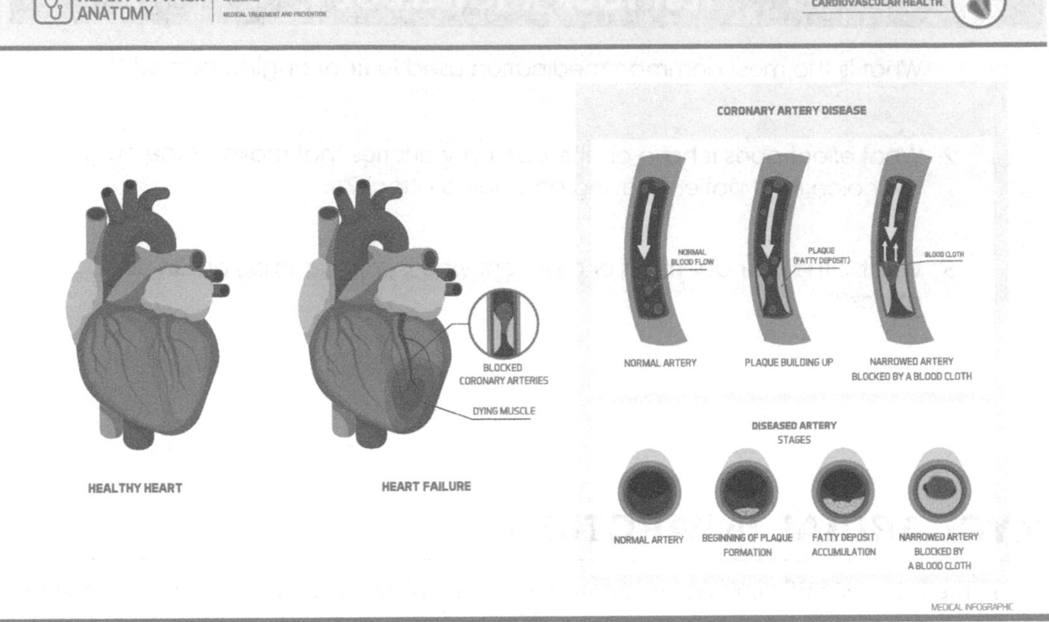

elenabsl/Shutterstock.com

FIGURE 11-6 The progression of coronary artery disease resulting in a myocardial infarction

Signs and Symptoms of a Myocardial Infarction

The pain associated with myocardial infarction most often occurs when the patient is at rest. When questioned after this type of episode, most patients report that they experienced angina-type pain hours to days prior to the myocardial infarction. The compressing, squeezing pain usually begins in the substernal area and then spreads to other areas. The pain associated with myocardial infarction may vary in degree from severe to almost nonexistent. It may last for 30 minutes or may even continue until analgesic medication is administered. This pain is not relieved by nitroglycerin.

Furthermore, while both men and women can experience any of these symptoms, woman are more likely to experience shortness of breath, abdomen pain, nausea, lightheadedness, vomiting, and neck and jaw pain. In the final stages, the patient may pass through stupor, coma, and ultimately death. A myocardial infarction, if not managed appropriately, can lead to cardiac arrest. See Emergency Basics 11-4 for a summary of the signs and symptoms of myocardial infarction.

Management of a Myocardial Infarction

Management of a myocardial infarction is outlined in Emergency Basics 11-5.

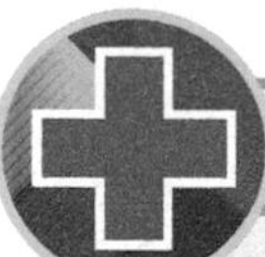

Emergency Basics 11-4

Signs and Symptoms of Myocardial Infarction

- Pain usually occurs at rest
- Compressing, squeezing pain beginning in substernal area and spreading
- Severity of pain varies
- Pain is not relieved by nitroglycerin
- Cold, clammy skin
- Dyspnea
- Vomiting
- Nausea
- Sweating
- Weakness or extreme fatigue
- Feeling of impending doom

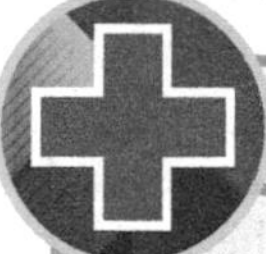

Emergency Basics 11-5

Management of Suspected Myocardial Infarction in the Dental Office

1. Remain calm.
2. Stop dental treatment.
3. Position patient upright as this is usually most comfortable.
4. Assess the situation, check circulation by palpation of the carotid artery, monitor breathing, and maintain an open airway.
5. Summon EMS to transport patient to hospital.
6. Administer morphine or nitrous oxide to alleviate pain.
7. Administer oxygen.
8. Administer 325 milligrams aspirin and ask patient to chew and swallow.
9. Record vital signs every 5 minutes.
10. Be prepared to perform BLS/CPR.

TEST YOUR KNOWLEDGE

1. What is a key event that will indicate to the dental team that the patient is experiencing more than angina pectoris?

2. How would the dental auxiliary position the patient if it is suspected that the patient is experiencing a myocardial infarction?

DENTAL MANAGEMENT OF THE PATIENT WITH A HISTORY OF A MYOCARDIAL INFARCTION

The dental health care provider will encounter patients with a history of myocardial infarction. A thorough medical history is important in identifying the patient with this history. The patient should be questioned regarding previous history of chest pain as well as a history of heart disease, diabetes, thyroid disorders, or adrenal gland disorders. Any previous hospitalizations as well as surgeries and medications should be noted in the patient's record. Medications the patient may be taking include any of the following: anticoagulants, daily aspirin to prevent clotting, **antihypertensive** medications, **diuretics**, nitroglycerine due to residual angina from the myocardial infarction, and cholesterol lowering medications. The patient's blood pressure should be recorded and evaluated for hypertension. If the patient confirms that they have a history of myocardial infarction, the dental health care provider should ask if there has been more than one and also when it occurred. A myocardial infarction usually results in residual damage to a portion of the heart muscle; part of the heart muscle dies and the remainder of the muscle must compensate for that part. A patient who has suffered from a myocardial infarction more than 6 months ago and has no residual complications from the infarct is an ASA II classification. A patient who has suffered from a myocardial infarction more than 6 months ago and has complications such as arrhythmias or **congestive heart failure** from the infarct is an ASA III classification depending on the severity of the complications. A patient who has had a myocardial infarction less than 6 months ago is not a candidate for elective care as the risk of a second myocardial infarction is high during this time. If urgent dental care is required, the patient should be treated in a hospital setting,

ANGINA AND MYOCARDIAL INFARCTION

Though angina and myocardial infarction have some differences, there are similarities as well. This section will discuss how the two can be differentiated.

Differences Between Angina and Myocardial Infarction

Being aware of the differences between angina and myocardial infarction will help the dental team in determining which one a patient is experiencing. These differences include the following:

- The pain associated with myocardial infarction is usually greater in severity and duration than with angina.
- A myocardial infarction, at times, may occur in the absence of physical exertion or emotional stress.
- The patient who is experiencing myocardial infarction continues to move about, trying to find a comfortable position, whereas the angina patient usually remains motionless.
- Nitroglycerine will not alleviate the pain of a myocardial Infarction.

TEST YOUR KNOWLEDGE

1. What are some medications that a patient with a previous history of a myocardial infarction may be taking?

2. How can the dental auxiliary tell the difference between a patient experiencing a myocardial infarction and a patient experiencing an angina attack?

SUMMARY

Heart disease is the leading cause of death in the United States today and is therefore a possible emergency the dental team may have to deal with. Angina is a condition most patients are aware that they have and will note on the health history. In these situations, the auxiliary and the dental team should do everything possible to alleviate undue stress, which may trigger an angina episode. It is certainly more beneficial to prevent an angina attack from occurring than to treat it once it happens. Angina, allowed to progress without proper treatment, may escalate to myocardial infarction. At the same time, myocardial infarction can occur without the patient having a history of angina. The dental team should try to prevent as much stress as possible and then be aware of the signs, symptoms, and treatment for a cardiac emergency in case it occurs while a patient is in the dental office.

REVIEW QUESTIONS

MULTIPLE CHOICE

1. Which layer of the wall of the heart gives the heart the ability to contract?
   a. epicardium
   b. myocardium
   c. endocardium
   d. pericardium

2. Which of the following is not a characteristic of unstable angina?
   a. Episodes may occur at rest
   b. No alteration in frequency
   c. May require higher dose of nitroglycerin
   d. Episodes often increase in intensity and duration

3. Which of the following is a precipitating factor of angina?
   a. drinking a cold drink
   b. sexual activity
   c. walking
   d. all the above

4. When managing patients experiencing an angina attack, why is it best to give the patients their own nitroglycerine?
   a. The office supply of nitroglycerin should be saved for patients who are not taking nitroglycerin
   b. You will be assured that the nitroglycerin has not expired
   c. The dosage will be adjusted for that particular patient
   d. None of the above

5. If all the steps of management for angina do not relieve the pain, the dental team should assume that the patient is suffering from which of the following?
   a. cerebrovascular accident
   b. cardiac arrest
   c. respiratory distress
   d. myocardial infarction

6. Which of the following is not correct regarding management of the dental patient with a history of angina?
   a. Diabetics are at a higher risk for an angina attack.
   b. It is not necessary for patients with a history of angina to bring their own nitroglycerine to the office.
   c. The patient with a history of angina may be taking an anticoagulant.
   d. It is important to review the medical history of the patient with a history of angina.

7. Which of the following is not a sign or symptom of myocardial infarction?
   a. Always occurs following physical exertion or emotional stress
   b. Compressing, squeezing pain in the substernal area
   c. May last in duration for 30 minutes or more
   d. A feeling of impending doom

8. When positioning the patient experiencing myocardial infarction, it is best to place the patient in which position?
   a. supine
   b. seated upright
   c. lying down
   d. none of the above

9. Which of the following defines the syndrome characterized by episodes of pain when the heart experiences oxygen deficiency?
   a. cardiac arrest
   b. myocardial infarction
   c. pulmonary edema
   d. angina pectoris

10. Which of the following is a sign or symptom of angina?
   a. substernal chest pain
   b. patient remains motionless
   c. increase in blood pressure
   d. all the above

TRUE OR FALSE

_______ 1. Atherosclerosis is the form of arteriosclerosis that affects the coronary arteries and causes coronary artery disease.

_______ 2. The amount of stress necessary to cause an angina attack can vary from time to time.

_______ 3. The most common symptom of angina is pain.

_______ 4. If a patient begins to experience angina in the dental office, there is no need to review the medical history.

_______ 5. Coronary artery disease does not progress in severity with time.

_______ 6. A patient who has suffered from a myocardial infarction more than 6 months ago and has complications such as arrhythmias or congestive heart failure from the infarct is an ASA II classification.

_______ 7. Nitroglycerin should be placed sublingually and allowed to dissolve.

_______ 8. Orthostatic hypotension is the only side effect of nitroglycerin.

_______ 9. Angina pectoris never advances to myocardial infarction.

_______ 10. Pain associated with myocardial infarction is usually relieved by nitroglycerin.

MEDICAL EMERGENCY!

CASE STUDY 11-1

A 44-year-old male presents with a positive medical history. He indicates on the medical history that he has been experiencing angina attacks for two years. He has his nitroglycerin with him. He is in the office to have an amalgam placed in tooth number 12. The dentist administers anesthesia and begins treatment. The patient becomes pale and starts to clutch at his chest. The dentist stops treatment and allows the patient to administer his own nitroglycerin. The patient says his chest pain is usually not so severe. He tries to get up and move around in an effort to relieve the pain. After several minutes, the patient's pain still has not been relieved. The patient takes another dose of nitroglycerin, but the pain still does not stop.

Questions

1. Is the patient most likely suffering from angina or myocardial infarction?

2. What management steps should be followed after administering the second dose of nitroglycerin?

3. Should oxygen be administered to this patient? Why or why not?

4. What should the dental auxiliary be doing during this treatment?

CASE STUDY 11-2

A 64-year-old male presents with a positive medical history. He states that he has had two heart attacks in the last two years. As the dental treatment begins, the dental auxiliary notes that the patient's skin has become cold and clammy. The patient reports a feeling of tightness in his chest.

Questions

1. Is the patient experiencing angina pectoris or a myocardial infarction? Explain your answer.
2. What medication should be given to this patient?
3. List the steps to manage this emergency.

SECTION FIVE

Immune System Emergencies

This section deals with localized and systemic medical conditions and emergencies that involve the immune system.

CHAPTER 12

Allergic Reactions

LEARNING OUTCOMES

Upon completion of this chapter, the student will be able to:

- Differentiate between an antigen and antibody
- Describe the functions of the immune system
- Explain what must take place for an allergic reaction to occur
- Explain the importance of a thorough medical history when treating a patient with allergies
- Explain the signs, symptoms, and management of allergic skin reactions
- Define an anaphylactic reaction
- Describe the signs and symptoms associated with an anaphylactic reaction
- Explain the management of an anaphylactic reaction
- Describe the role of epinephrine in managing allergic reactions
- Determine a true allergy to dental anesthesia
- List the signs and symptoms associated with latex allergy
- Describe the protocol to follow when a staff member or patient is allergic to latex

KEY TERMS

anaphylaxis
angioedema
antibody
antigen
cardiac arrhythmias
contact dermatitis
edema
engulf
erythema
immune system
immunoglobulin system
interferons
latex allergy
lymphocytes
neoprene
phagocytes
shock
urticaria
vesicle

INTRODUCTION

A vast majority of the population is allergic to one thing or another. The reaction to this allergy may range from a slight rash and runny nose to a fatal anaphylactic reaction. To understand an allergic reaction, it is important to understand the functions and makeup of the body's **immune system**. The immune system is highly complex and designed to protect us from the millions of microorganisms and other invaders we face every day. However, that protective mechanism can become life threatening if the body's immune system responds to an invader through a heightened allergic response.

THE IMMUNE SYSTEM

This section will discuss the importance of antibodies and their role in the immune system response when an antigen invades.

Antigens

An **antigen**, sometimes called an *allergen,* is a substance that enters the body and can produce a hypersensitive reaction but is not necessarily intrinsically harmful. Most people develop a natural or acquired immunity to allergens, but in people who suffer from allergies, the body is overly sensitive to the antigen. When an allergic reaction occurs, the body's immune system is not protecting itself against the allergen.

Physiologic Defense

Regardless of the severity of the allergic reaction, the underlying chemical and physiological aspects are similar. The body has a variety of defense mechanisms that prevent the entry of an antigen. The first line of defense used by the body is a form of barriers. One barrier, skin (the largest organ in the body), prevents entry of various antigens we come across every second of every day. A cut or an open wound may allow passage of the antigen into the body. Another defense mechanism is the lining of the nasal passages. The lining contains tiny hairs called *cilia* that trap particles and prevent their entry into the airways. In the event that the first line of defense is unable to prevent entry of the antigen into the body, the second line of defense becomes active.

The second line of defense includes body chemicals and cellular activities. **Interferons** are proteins produced by infected cells. They are released to other cells causing noninfected cells to produce proteins that prevent the virus from invading and replicating. Approximately 20 other body chemicals also destroy various antigens. A specialized white blood cell, known as a natural killer cell, may also become activated by the presence of an antigen, resulting in destruction of that antigen. **Phagocytes** may activate to **engulf** the antigen (Figure 12-1). Once engulfed, it is then destroyed by the chemicals present in the phagocyte.

If an antigen manages to escape any of these defense mechanisms, a specific response mechanism involving the immune system is activated. The bone marrow, spleen, thymus, and lymph nodes produce cells important in this specific immune response. The unique feature of this particular system is that it has memory.

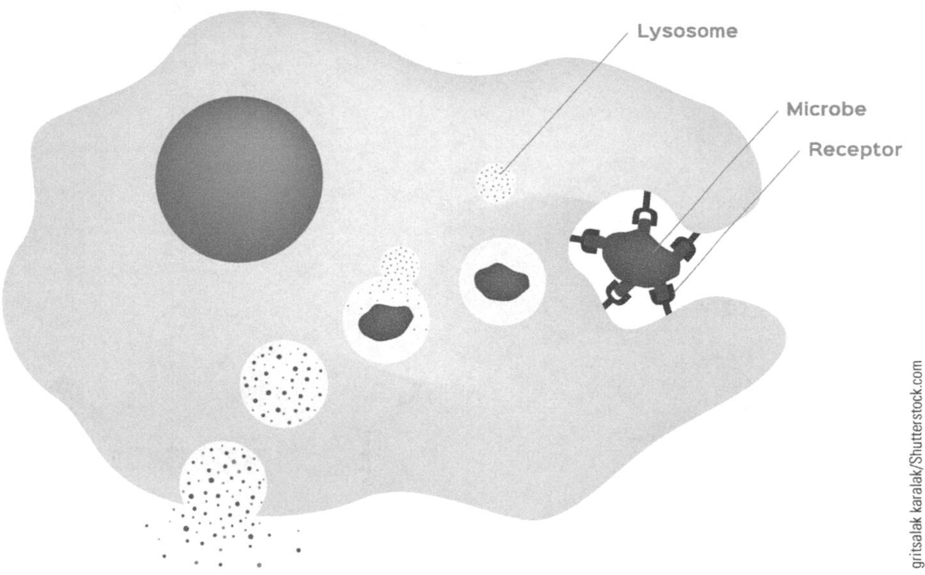

FIGURE 12-1 Phagocytosis of a foreign pathogen is activated

Several types of white blood cells form this part of specific immune response. The B **lymphocytes** are the major force of this memory specific immune system and are produced by the bone marrow, though they spend quite a bit of time in the lymphatic fluid. Another cell, known as the T lymphocyte, is also produced in the bone marrow. The T cells destroy the antigen once it has been identified by the antibodies. A third type of specialized white cell is the macrophage, which will "clean up" the remains of the antigen destroyed due to the specific immune response.

Antibodies

B cells produce antibodies or proteins that are specific to an antigen and result in its destruction. An **antibody** is an essential part of the body's immune system. Antibodies are produced when a virus, bacteria, or another foreign substance enters the body. A particular type of antibody is produced for each foreign substance, which is called an *allergen* or *antigen*. So far, five different classifications of antibodies have been discovered. Together they make up the **immunoglobulin system**. Refer to Figure 12-2.

Immunoglobulin A (IgA) antibodies are found in areas of the body such as the nose, breathing passages, digestive tract, ears, eyes, and vagina. IgA antibodies protect body surfaces that are exposed to outside foreign substances. This type of antibody is also found in saliva, tears, and blood. IgA is found in all the secretions of the body and helps protect the body from dangerous microorganisms.

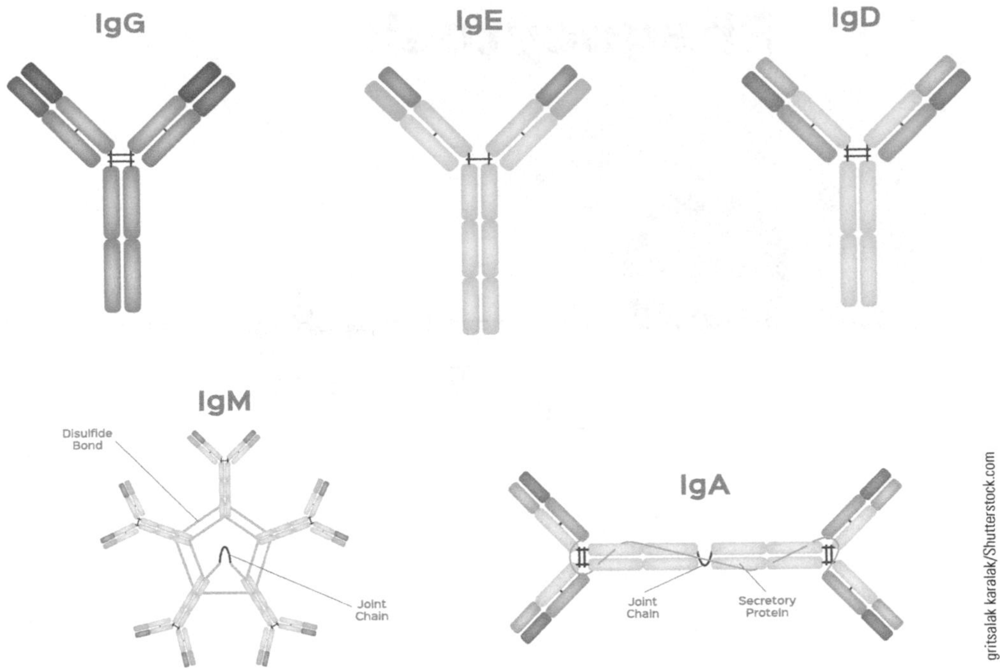

FIGURE 12-2 The five antibodies making up the immunoglobulin system

Immunoglobulin D (IgD) antibodies are found in small amounts in the tissues that line the belly or chest and in serum tissue. The precise function of the IgD antibody has not been determined.

Immunoglobulin E (IgE) antibodies are found in the lungs, skin, and mucous membranes. They cause the body to react against foreign substances such as pollen, fungus spores, and animal dander. They may occur in allergic reactions to milk, some medicines, and some poisons. IgE antibody levels are often high in people with allergies and are responsible for reacting with certain antigens and causing type I reactions, which are anaphylactic reactions.

Immunoglobulin G (IgG) antibodies are found in all body fluids. They are the smallest but most common antibody. IgG antibodies are important in fighting bacterial and viral infections. IgG antibodies are the only type of antibody that can cross the placenta in a pregnant woman to help protect the fetus.

Immunoglobulin M (IgM) antibodies are the largest antibody. They are found in blood and lymph fluid and are the first type of antibody made in response to an infection or exposure to a foreign antigen.

PREREQUISITES FOR ALLERGIC REACTIONS

A person does not experience an allergic reaction during the first exposure to the antigen. For example, a person who is going to be allergic to penicillin does not experience any reaction the first time the drug is given. This first dose is known as the sensitizing dose. After this dose, the body produces the IgE antibody, which reacts only to this particular antigen. For a period after exposure, the IgE antibody continues to be produced while the antigen decreases. After a certain time, only the specific IgE antibody is circulating in the body. At this point no allergic reaction occurs.

When the person is exposed again to this same allergen, or one that is chemically similar, an allergic reaction does occur. This results as the body recognizes the antigen, and biochemical elements that cause the reaction are released. The main biochemical element is histamine. Histamine is found in all cells but is only released in allergic reactions. It has the ability to cause dilation of the capillaries, increased secretion of the gastric juices, decreased blood pressure, and constriction of some of the smooth muscles. The type of allergic reaction that results depends mainly on the type and amount of allergen involved.

IMPORTANCE OF MEDICAL HISTORY

Medical history is especially important when treating an allergy-prone patient. It has been determined that a person with a history of allergies to several substances (such as pollen, eggs, seafood, and penicillin) is likely to experience an allergic reaction to some item or drug used in the dental office. This person's body responses are highly sensitized, and the patient requires special attention during dental procedures.

In addition, medical history is important in telling the dental staff what substances have actually caused the patient to experience an allergic reaction. For example, if a patient reports experience in the past of an allergic reaction to a particular agent used in the dental office, the dental team would not use this item during the procedure.

TEST YOUR KNOWLEDGE

1. What is the immunoglobulin that is responsible for causing type I reactions?
2. What are the effects of histamine on the patient's tissue?
3. What is the most important item that a dental auxiliary can obtain from a patient that will prevent allergic reactions?

TYPES OF ALLERGIC REACTIONS

Allergic reactions vary in type and severity. The reaction may occur almost immediately because of the humoral system or may be delayed for several days as a result of the cell-mediated system. The reaction may be localized to one area, such as a skin reaction, or may be generalized, involving the whole body, as in an anaphylactic reaction. Refer to Figure 12-3. In the 1970s, two scientists, P. G. H. Gell and R. A. Coombs, came up with a classification system that differentiates the four types of hypersensitivity reactions. See Emergency Basics 12-1 for a summary of this classification.

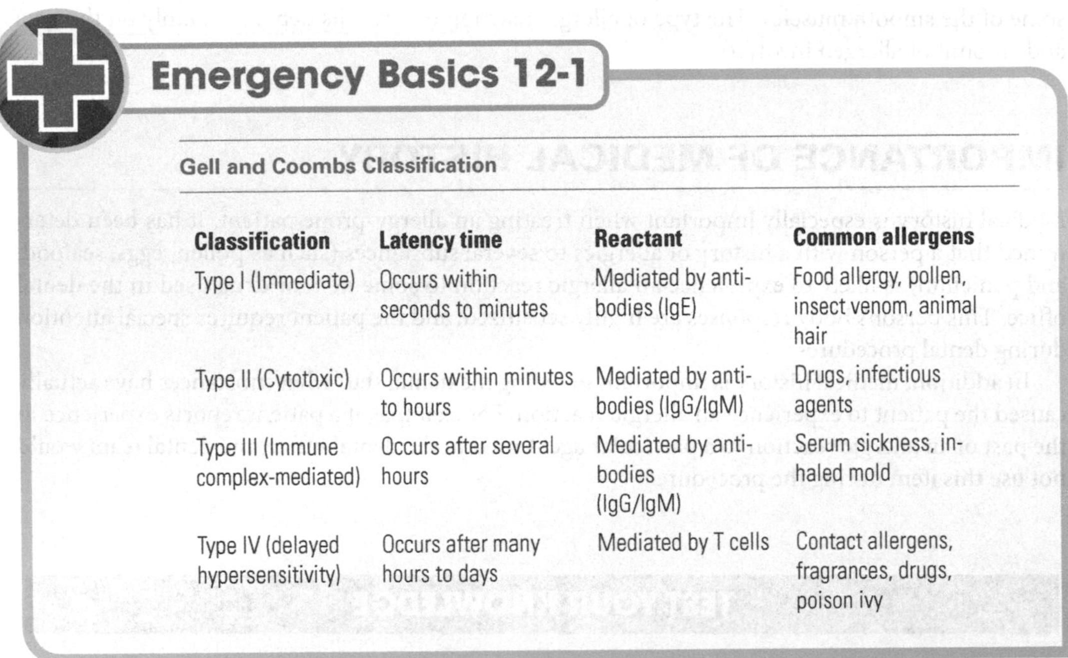

Emergency Basics 12-1

Gell and Coombs Classification

Classification	Latency time	Reactant	Common allergens
Type I (Immediate)	Occurs within seconds to minutes	Mediated by antibodies (IgE)	Food allergy, pollen, insect venom, animal hair
Type II (Cytotoxic)	Occurs within minutes to hours	Mediated by antibodies (IgG/IgM)	Drugs, infectious agents
Type III (Immune complex-mediated)	Occurs after several hours	Mediated by antibodies (IgG/IgM)	Serum sickness, inhaled mold
Type IV (delayed hypersensitivity)	Occurs after many hours to days	Mediated by T cells	Contact allergens, fragrances, drugs, poison ivy

In some instances, it is possible to predetermine the severity of a reaction. The time that elapses between exposure to the allergen and the onset of the allergic reaction determines to a great extent the severity of the reaction. If some reaction is noticed within a few minutes of exposure, the reaction may be much more severe than when the reaction is seen several hours to a few days after the exposure.

Skin Reactions

There is a wide variety of skin disorders, ranging from mild to severe. Skin reactions may also be the first stage of anaphylactic reactions. No matter how mild the skin reaction seems, the progression of a skin reaction should be watched carefully. The more quickly a skin reaction occurs, the greater the likelihood that the allergic reaction will progress into a serious reaction that may involve the airway.

Contact Dermatitis

Contact dermatitis is an allergic skin reaction that occurs as a result of cutaneous exposure to a particular allergen and may occur in the oral mucosa as well as in the skin. The allergen that causes

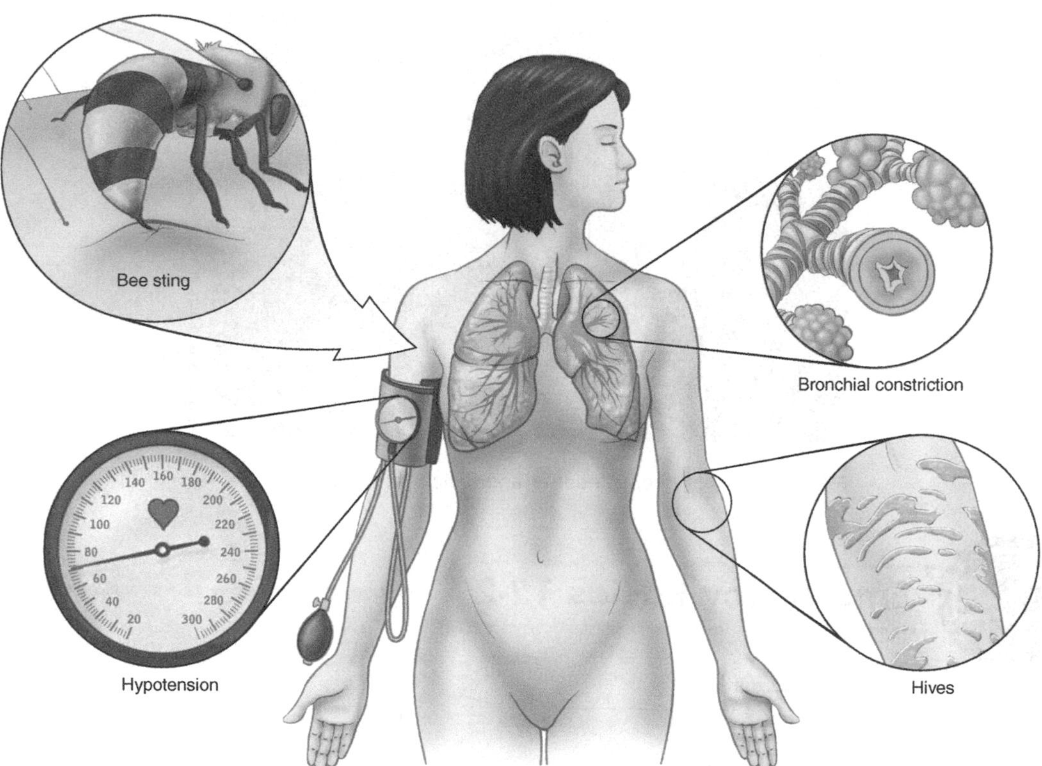

FIGURE 12-3 Allergic reactions vary greatly in type and severity. Reactions can manifest in a range from skin reactions, such as urticaria (commonly known as hives), to extreme cases such as laryngeal edema (swelling of the larynx) due to an anaphylactic allergic reaction. All allergic reactions require prompt treatment.
Source: Ehrlich, 9781305634435, Medical Terminology for Health Professions 8e, Figure 6-7

this type of reaction may include such items as poison ivy, toothpaste, mouthwash, lipstick or other cosmetics, impression materials, metal alloys, and stainless-steel wire. Contact dermatitis is usually an acute problem, but if the allergen is not removed and exposure continues, the condition becomes chronic and in some cases disabling.

The first signs of contact dermatitis include **erythema** (redness), **edema** (swelling), and **vesicle** (blister) formation (Figure 12-4). In some serious cases these vesicles may rupture and result in open, oozing wounds. The main symptom is intense itching. This symptom, as well as the condition, is usually localized to the one area where the antigen contacted the surface, although in a few cases it may spread.

In most cases, the first step of management of the allergic reaction is to remove the contacting substance. A physician may further administer corticosteroids and antihistamines.

See Emergency Basics 12-2 for a summary of the signs/symptoms and management of contact dermatitis.

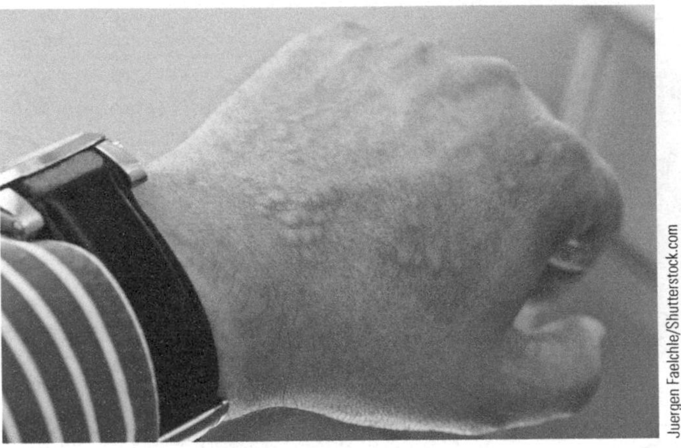

FIGURE 12-4 Erythema, edema, and vesicle formation

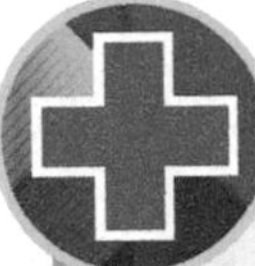

Emergency Basics 12-2

Contact Dermatitis

Signs and Symptoms
- Itching
- Erythema
- Edema
- Vesicle formation

Management
- Remove source of allergen
- Administer antihistamine
- Administer corticosteroids

Urticaria

Urticaria is a skin condition most of the general public calls hives (see Figure 12-5). It may be caused by any substance that is either ingested or placed on the skin surface. This condition consists of circumscribed raised areas of erythema and edema, and as with any allergic reaction, it may be mild or severe.

As with contact dermatitis, the main course of management is to remove the substance. The patient may be given instructions to take an over-the-counter antihistamine. If the symptoms persist, the patient may need to contact a physician. For example, if the urticaria was caused by some substance that the patient ingested, the course of management would be to stop the ingestion of the substance.

See Emergency Basics 12-3 for a summary of the signs/symptoms and management of urticaria.

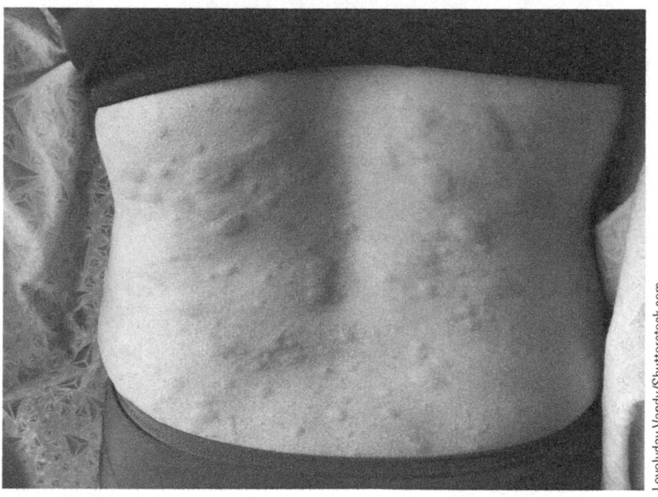

Lovelyday Vandy/Shutterstock.com

FIGURE 12-5 Urticaria on the back

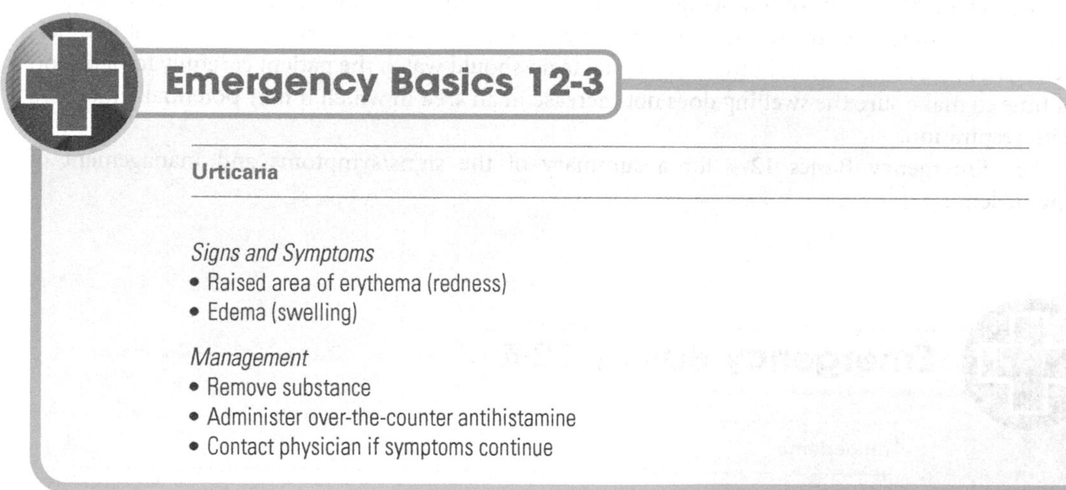

Emergency Basics 12-3

Urticaria

Signs and Symptoms

- Raised area of erythema (redness)
- Edema (swelling)

Management

- Remove substance
- Administer over-the-counter antihistamine
- Contact physician if symptoms continue

Angioedema

In its beginning stages, **angioedema**, also called *angioneurotic edema*, is sometimes mistaken for urticaria. Basically, angioedema is a larger form of urticaria. It is characterized by localized swelling of either the submucosa or subcutaneous tissues (Figure 12-6). The lesions associated with angioedema have certain characteristics: usually the lesions are single, but in some cases they may be multiple; they are large and do not have defined raised borders like urticaria; and there is no pain and usually no associated itching. The tissues of the genitals, face, and hands are the areas usually affected by angioedema.

Angioedema is usually caused by an allergic reaction to drugs, food, or environmental factors. As with most skin reactions, angioedema occurs when an antigen enters the body, histamine is released, capillaries dilate, and fluid enters the area. It is commonly seen in people with a history of various allergies but may also be found in those with no allergy history.

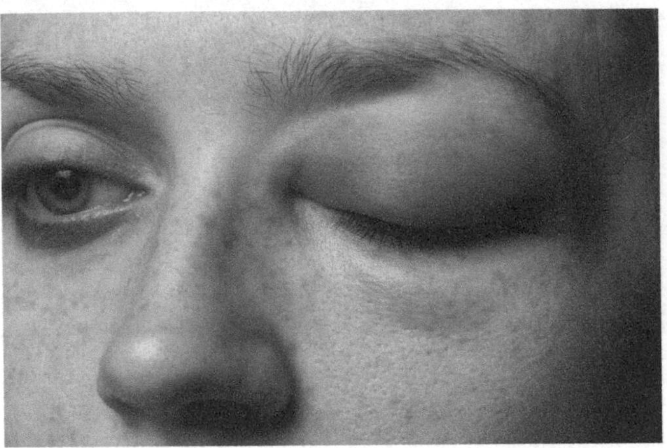

Chris Tefme/Shutterstock.com

FIGURE 12-6 Angioedema

Management consists of removing the cause and administering an antihistamine. In most cases these steps will reverse the situation without major complications occurring. However, if the incident takes place in the dental office, the dental team should watch the patient carefully for a period of time to make sure the swelling does not increase in an area in which it may potentially interfere with respiration.

See Emergency Basics 12-4 for a summary of the signs/symptoms and management of angioedema.

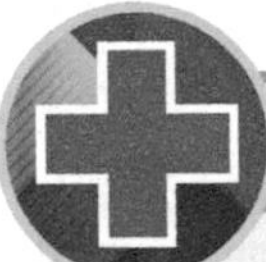

Emergency Basics 12-4

Angioedema

Signs and Symptoms

- Localized swelling of submucosa
- Localized swelling of subcutaneous tissue
- Usually single lesions
- No pain
- No itching

Management

- Remove the cause
- Administer antihistamine

Note that in most mild cases of allergic skin reactions, the dentist may choose not to treat the patient in the dental office but rather refer the patient to a physician or allergist. This action may prove satisfactory, but the dental team should observe the patient and always provide follow-up management either in the office or by referral.

Most skin reactions do not create emergency situations in themselves. The major cause for concern is that skin reactions may either advance and create an emergency or be the beginning of a true emergency situation such as anaphylactic shock.

TEST YOUR KNOWLEDGE

1. Which type of allergic reaction occurs as a result of direct exposure to an allergen?
2. What areas of the body are most often affected by angioedema?
3. In general, what is the management for most allergic reactions in a dental office?

Respiratory Allergic Reactions

Allergic reactions that may affect only the respiratory system also occur. The most common type of respiratory reaction, asthma, is discussed in detail in Chapter 8.

ANAPHYLACTIC REACTION

An anaphylactic reaction is a severe allergic reaction that occurs in previously sensitized patients. It develops almost immediately after the patient ingests, inhales, or is injected with an antigen or is stung by an insect. **Anaphylaxis** is the most severe allergic reaction and can prove fatal if not managed quickly.

Physiology

As with other allergic reactions, anaphylaxis occurs only in those who have been previously exposed to the allergen. The patient is exposed to the allergen, an incubation period then takes place, and antibodies form. When the patient is exposed to the same allergen, the anaphylactic reaction occurs. This is sometimes called the exciting or shock dose, which is how the name anaphylactic shock came into existence.

Severity

Symptoms associated with anaphylaxis can vary in a wide range of severity that depends on the amount of acquired sensitivity, the amount of antigen that entered the body, and the method in which the antigen entered the body. Furthermore, the time that elapses between the exposure to the antigen and the onset of symptoms usually indicates how serious the reaction will be. For example, reactions that occur within the first 30 minutes after contact with the antigen are usually the most severe. Reactions that occur after 30 minutes are less likely to be fatal.

Symptoms

Signs and symptoms associated with anaphylaxis vary in both type and severity. These may be seen in the skin, gastrointestinal, respiratory, or circulatory systems. A common term used to describe these signs and symptoms is **shock.**

Shock is best described as a decrease in perfusion of oxygenated blood to the organs in the body. This condition can be the result of a physical trauma or, in the case of allergies, a release of chemicals that diminish the ability of the cardiac and pulmonary systems to supply oxygenated blood. As a result, the organs of the body begin to fail and toxins are produced that increase the signs and symptoms reported in a patient experiencing shock.

Signs and symptoms associated with the skin in allergic reactions may include generalized pruritus (itching), urticaria, or angioedema. Normally these conditions are not too dangerous, but they do have the potential to become life-threatening if they are located in some specific areas. For example, angioedema located around the mouth or throat could cause death from airway obstruction. Gastrointestinal signs and symptoms may include nausea, vomiting, and diarrhea.

Respiratory signs and symptoms may include varying degrees of airway obstruction. This most often occurs as a result of laryngeal edema, a swelling of the larynx that occurs as a result of an allergic reaction (see Figure 12-3). The swelling may be great enough to cause partial or even complete obstruction of the airway. It is the most common cause of death in anaphylactic reactions.

Circulatory signs and symptoms may include hypotension, shock, **cardiac arrhythmias**, and even complete circulatory collapse.

All the signs and symptoms associated with an anaphylactic reaction vary in their severity as well as in the way they present themselves. Nevertheless, diagnosis can be relatively easy if the signs and symptoms occur right after the exposure. In this situation, almost immediately the patient will feel faint and weak, will begin sweating, and will become anxious and restless. The patient then develops a severe itching sensation as a result of allergic skin reactions. The condition then proceeds through the gastrointestinal, respiratory, and circulatory stages. If this cycle is not stopped, the end result will be death.

See Emergency Basics 12-5 for a summary of the signs and symptoms of anaphylaxis.

Dental Management of the Patient with an Allergic Reaction

At the first sign of an anaphylactic reaction, place the patient in a supine position and administer oxygen. The receptionist should summon emergency medical assistance. In the meantime, the dental auxiliary should retrieve the emergency kit and prepare an epinephrine injection; the dentist should administer the epinephrine immediately. Remember that a subsequent injection of epinephrine may be required. If more than one injection of epinephrine is needed, the dentist may also administer an injection of antihistamine during the acute phase.

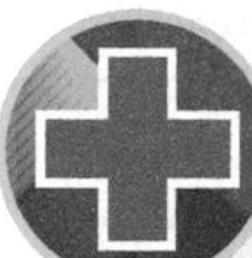

Emergency Basics 12-5

Signs and Symptoms of Anaphylaxis

Skin
- Generalized pruritus (itching)
- Urticaria
- Angioedema

Gastrointestinal
- Nausea
- Vomiting
- Diarrhea

Respiratory
- Laryngeal edema

Circulatory
- Hypotension
- Shock
- Cardiac arrhythmias
- Complete circulatory collapse

Additional Symptoms
- Sweating
- Anxious feeling
- Nervousness

During the entire episode, attention must be paid to the patient's airway, since laryngeal edema may cause the airway to become blocked. However, once the epinephrine is administered, the patient's condition should improve. If laryngeal edema occurs and complete airway obstruction results, the dental auxiliary should be prepared to assist the dentist in performing a cricothyrotomy (Refer back to Chapter 10). If there is a complete loss of blood pressure and/or pulse, the dentist and auxiliary should begin cardiopulmonary resuscitation (CPR) until medical assistance arrives.

The management just described is specific for an anaphylactic reaction that demonstrates the signs and symptoms mentioned earlier. A unique problem with the anaphylactic reaction is that, in some cases, the reaction is so severe that the signs and symptoms occur quickly and seem to happen all at once. In this situation, the patient may become unconscious almost immediately, and it may be difficult to determine that the condition was caused by an allergic reaction.

When there are no definitive signs of an allergic reaction, the dentist should not administer epinephrine. Instead, the patient should be placed in the Trendelenburg position, basic life support provided as needed with extra attention paid to maintaining the airway, and emergency medical assistance summoned. If the condition worsens, CPR or cricothyrotomy may become necessary.

The dental team can administer oxygen to a patient suspected of having an allergic reaction. Oxygen administered through a nasal cannula or face mask will not harm the patient or make the reaction worse.

See Emergency Basics 12-6 for a summary of the management of anaphylaxis both for patients with obvious signs and symptoms and for patients with whom it is not clear whether an allergic reaction has caused the condition.

EPINEPHRINE

In the management of severe allergic reactions, epinephrine is the drug of choice. Epinephrine is a vasopressor, has antihistaminic action, and is a bronchodilator (Figure 12-7). Its effect is extremely rapid in onset. This characteristic in particular makes it especially useful in the management of anaphylactic reactions when time is crucial.

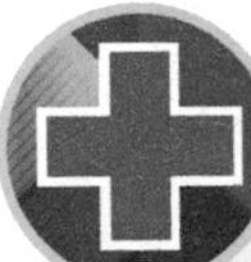

Emergency Basics 12-6

Management of Anaphylaxis

Patient with Obvious Signs and Symptoms

1. Summon medical assistance
2. Place the patient in a supine position
3. Administer oxygen
4. Administer epinephrine
5. Administer antihistamine as needed
6. Initiate CPR if needed
7. Assist dentist in performing cricothyrotomy if necessary

Patient Without Signs or Symptoms

1. Summon medical assistance
2. Do not administer epinephrine
3. Place patient in Trendelenburg position
4. Provide basic life support as needed
5. Administer oxygen
6. Initiate CPR if needed
7. Assist dentist in performing cricothyrotomy if necessary

Although epinephrine is extremely beneficial in the management of allergic reactions, it should never be administered unless you are sure that the patient is suffering from an allergic reaction. Some conditions, such as cerebrovascular accident, may at first be mistaken for an allergic reaction, since the patient may lose consciousness. In such situations, administering epinephrine, which increases blood pressure, could cause extreme harm.

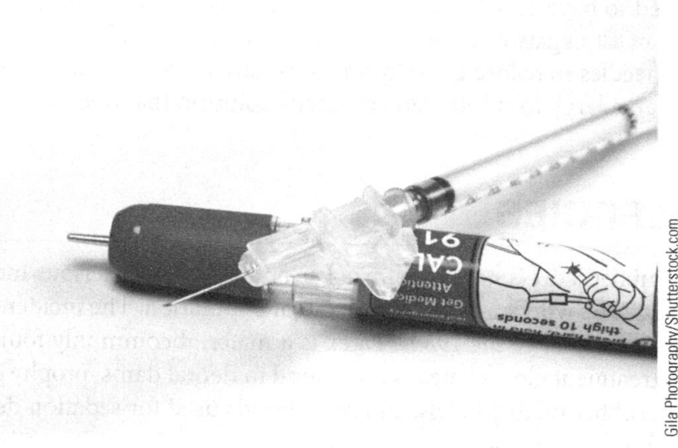

Gila Photography/Shutterstock.com

FIGURE 12-7 In severe allergic reactions, epinephrine is the drug used to rapidly reverse the symptoms of anaphylactic shock. It is of utmost importance to confirm that the patient is suffering an allergic reaction, and not another medical emergency, before administering epinephrine.

TEST YOUR KNOWLEDGE

1. What is the most common cause of death in a patient exhibiting signs of anaphylaxis?
2. Why should a dentist not administer epinephrine to a patient without being certain that the patient is experiencing an allergic reaction?
3. What is meant by the term *shock*?

ALLERGY TO DENTAL LOCAL ANESTHESIA

One aspect of allergic reactions unique to dentistry is an allergic reaction to dental anesthetic solutions. However, if a patient reports an allergy to dental anesthesia on the medical history, the dentist should explore the subject a little further. A true allergy to an amide local anesthetic is rare. If the patient reports an allergy, ask them about the type of reaction they experienced. If necessary, the patient may need to have an allergy test to confirm a true allergy. It has been estimated that less than 1 percent of all negative reactions to anesthesia are actually allergic reactions. Patients who are fearful of needles may lose consciousness usually before the anesthetic is administered. If a patient reports an allergy to sulfites, an anesthetic solution that does not contain epinephrine must be used.

LATEX ALLERGIES

Allergy to natural rubber latex is now recognized as an increasingly serious medical problem that affects not only health care workers but also the general population. The incidence of **latex allergies** has increased dramatically since the 1980s. Latex is a material commonly found in the dental office. In addition to treatment gloves, latex is also found in dental dams, prophy cups, dental tubing, stethoscope tubing, rubber mixing bowls, and nasal hoods used for sedation dentistry. There is an increased trend to eliminate the use of latex as much as possible. As an alternative, nitrile, vinyl, and **neoprene** gloves are available. Nasal hoods for sedation dentistry and dental dams are also available in a nonlatex alternative. Dental tubing can be purchased in a nonlatex form, and prophy cups are available also as a plastic rather than latex.

Allergic reactions to latex can range from minor skin irritations to fatal anaphylactic reactions. Because the minor skin reactions mimic so many common situations, they are often overlooked by the individual or even misdiagnosed by physicians.

Individuals at Risk for Latex Hypersensitivity

Both individuals with a genetic history of allergies and individuals with a high exposure to latex products are at an increased risk for latex hypersensitivity. In these instances, the risk tends to increase with greater exposure. Some studies have stated that 8 to 12 percent of health care workers with regular exposure to latex are sensitized, as compared to 1 to 6 percent of the general public. These percentages, especially with regard to health care workers, continue to increase.

Additional risk factors may include a history of surgery, disorders requiring repeated urinary catheterization, and certain food allergies including bananas, avocados, chestnuts, and kiwi.

Although a high incidence of latex allergies occurs in health care workers, a dental office must be prepared to deal with patients with this same allergy.

Signs and Symptoms of Latex Hypersensitivity

Three different types of reactions may be seen in individuals who are allergic to latex. The two most common reactions from exposure to latex products are contact dermatitis (see Figure 12-8) or a delayed contact reaction. Contact dermatitis may result in dry, itchy, irritated areas of the skin, usually the hands. A delayed contact reaction is similar to a poison ivy reaction. It typically occurs 48 to 72 hours after exposure and may include a red, itchy rash or possibly blisters.

The third type of reaction to latex exposure is the immediate allergic reaction. The signs of this reaction usually occur 2 to 3 minutes after contact with the latex. In this situation, the

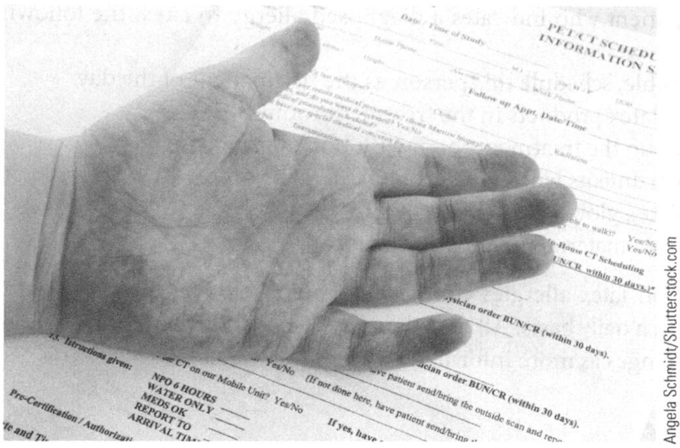

Angela Schmidt/Shutterstock.com

FIGURE 12-8 Contact dermatitis from a latex glove

individual may experience itching at the area of contact followed by welts or rash. These signs may disappear within 30 minutes. Additional immediate reactions may occur in individuals with sensitivity to airborne allergens associated with latex. This is commonly associated with powder used with latex gloves. This powder can be released as a result of putting on or removing gloves as well as by removing gloves from the glove box. The latex particles attach themselves to the powder and become airborne. As a result, sensitized individuals may experience coughing, wheezing, shortness of breath, and respiratory distress. The severity of the reaction depends on the sensitivity of the individual. In extreme cases, where sensitivity is extremely high, an anaphylactic reaction may occur.

Management

Currently there is no cure for latex allergy. Prevention and avoidance of exposure to latex and management of symptoms are the main options.

Should one of the three types of allergic reactions to latex exposure occur in a staff member or a patient, the management discussed in the previous sections of this chapter should be provided.

Prevention and Dental Management

Individuals must be tested by a physician to determine that they have a true allergy to latex. In individuals in which a true latex allergy has been diagnosed, protocols should be taken to prevent or minimize exposure to latex.

To minimize exposure to latex, sensitized dental staff members should do the following:

- Use nonlatex gloves and products.
- Learn to recognize the signs and symptoms of latex allergy.
- Avoid areas where powder from latex gloves worn by others might be inhaled.
- Inform employer and staff of the allergy.
- Wear a medical alert bracelet.

When treating a patient who indicates a diagnosed allergy to latex, the following steps should be implemented:

- When possible, schedule this person as the first patient of the day.
- Do not use latex products in the treatment room.
- Prepare/set up the treatment room with nonlatex gloves.
- Handle instruments with nonlatex gloves.
- Wear nonlatex gloves during treatment.
- Use latex-free materials and instruments.

New information on latex allergies continues to be developed. New products that are latex-free enter the market on a daily basis. All dental professionals should continue to seek education on this topic and make changes as more information becomes available.

SUMMARY

Allergic reactions in the dental office can be serious. The amount of management the auxiliary is allowed to perform, although not lacking in importance, is somewhat limited. Since the main method of management in severe reactions is an injection of epinephrine, the treatment must be performed by the dentist. It is nevertheless important for the auxiliary to understand what takes place during a reaction and assist the dentist by having all drugs prepared. Remember, in an anaphylactic reaction, death can occur quickly if correct steps are not taken. The auxiliary should also help the dentist administer CPR if this becomes necessary. A competent and calm team will make the management progress efficiently and professionally, which will benefit the well-being and health of the patient.

REVIEW QUESTIONS

MULTIPLE CHOICE

1. Which of the following is correct regarding the immune system?
   a. Antibody is also known as an allergen.
   b. Antigens are a major line of defense against allergens that enter the body.
   c. T cells destroy the antigen once it has been identified.
   d. Immunoglobulin E can cross the placenta and protect the fetus.

2. What is the foreign substance that enters the body and causes an allergic reaction?
   a. antibody
   b. lymph cell
   c. immunoglobulin
   d. antigen

3. Which type of allergic skin reaction occurs as a result of direct exposure of the skin to a/an particular allergen?
   a. contact dermatitis
   b. angioedema
   c. urticaria
   d. laryngeal edema

4. Which allergic skin reaction is also known as hives?
   a. contact dermatitis
   b. angioedema
   c. urticaria
   d. laryngeal edema

5. What is included in the management of angioedema?
   a. removing the cause
   b. administering an antibiotic
   c. administering an antihistamine
   d. a and c

6. Which of the following is not a characteristic of epinephrine?
   a. bronchoconstriction
   b. vasopressor
   c. reverses laryngeal edema
   d. has antihistaminic action

7. The most important part of managing an anaphylactic reaction consists of administering which of the following?
   a. oxygen
   b. antihistamine
   c. corticosteroid
   d. epinephrine

8. What is the most common cause of death associated with an anaphylactic reaction?
   a. hypotension
   b. laryngeal edema
   c. cardiovascular collapse
   d. none of the above

9. Which of the following is a function of histamine?
   a. dilation of the capillaries
   b. secretion of gastric juices
   c. decreased blood pressure
   d. all the above

10. Which of the following areas of the body are most often affected by angioedema?
    (1) torso
    (2) hands
    (3) face
    (4) genitals
    a. 1, 2, 3, 4
    b. 1, 2, 4
    c. 2, 3, 4
    d. 2, 3

TRUE OR FALSE

_______ 1. True allergies to local anesthetics are common.

_______ 2. A patient usually experiences an allergic reaction on first exposure to the harmful antigen.

_______ 3. The time that elapses between exposure to an antigen and the onset of symptoms helps in determining the severity of the upcoming reaction.

_______ 4. The patient with a history of allergies to several things is a likely candidate for an allergic reaction in the dental office.

_______ 5. The main symptom of contact dermatitis is swelling.

_______ 6. It is not uncommon for a person to die from a severe anaphylactic reaction even if proper management is provided.

_______ 7. Signs and symptoms associated with an anaphylactic reaction may be seen in the skin, gastrointestinal, respiratory, or circulatory system.

_______ 8. The signs and symptoms of an anaphylactic reaction never occur so rapidly that they cannot be distinguished.

_______ 9. A dentist who is not sure that the patient is suffering from an anaphylactic reaction should not administer epinephrine.

_______ 10. Patients who state they once experienced an allergic reaction to dental anesthesia should be evaluated by an allergist.

MEDICAL EMERGENCY!

CASE STUDY 12-1

A new dental assistant joins the office. One week after starting, she reports a "rash" on her hands. Her hands are itchy, irritated, and dry. There is no prior such occurrence based on what the dental assistant reports.

Questions

1. What is the cause of this reaction?

2. Should epinephrine be administered?

3. What should the office do to manage this problem going forward?

CASE STUDY 12-2

A 21-year-old male presents with a negative medical history and reports to be in good general health. The treatment planned for today is a tooth-colored restoration on a maxillary first molar. As the auxiliary is placing a latex dental dam, the patient begins to complain of itching around his lips. No previous reaction has been noted in the treatment record.

Questions

1. What is the most likely cause of the itching?

2. What should be the first step in managing this patient?

3. What notation should be placed in the patient's medical history update?

SECTION SIX

Legal Issues in Emergency Care

This section deals with the legal issues that are a part of emergency treatment.

CHAPTER 13

Occupational Hazards and Emergencies

LEARNING OUTCOMES

Upon completion of this chapter, the student will be able to:

- Explain the hazards of mercury contamination
- Explain how to prevent mercury contamination
- Describe how to avoid the hazards of ionizing radiation
- Describe universal precautions and PPE
- Describe how to prevent breakage of an anesthetic needle
- Explain the treatment for a broken endodontic file or reamer
- Explain how the auxiliary can help prevent soft-tissue injuries
- Describe the hazards of nitrous oxide/oxygen conscious sedation

KEY TERMS

anxiolytic
endodontic file
endodontic reamer
ionizing radiation
personal protective equipment (PPE)
titration
universal precautions

Most emergencies in the dental office occur as a result of some associated medical condition. These emergencies can occur with a patient or a member of the dental office team. However, some emergencies may take place as a result of the dental treatment itself, and there are conditions in the dental office that present hazards to the dental personnel as well.

The first section of this chapter covers hazards present in the dental office that have the potential to injure office personnel. The second section presents a few of the more common emergencies that can arise as a result of certain dental procedures.

HAZARDS TO OFFICE PERSONNEL

A number of potential hazards can directly or indirectly affect the dental auxiliary. However, when hazardous conditions or materials are properly handled, most of these risks can be minimized significantly.

Mercury Contamination

The use of amalgam as a restorative material has diminished as a result of the improvement of tooth-colored restorative materials. However, amalgam still remains in use as a restorative material because of its strength and durability. Since one of the major components of amalgam is mercury, the dental auxiliary should be aware of the potentially toxic effects of mercury poisoning. Although mercury has potential for causing serious problems within the dental office, if handled properly, it need not be an occupational hazard.

Mercury can be absorbed through the skin if the auxiliary handles it improperly during the preparation of amalgam. However, mercury is absorbed mainly by inhalation of vapors in the air. Mercury vapors can be released into the air by improperly storing scrap amalgam, by spilling mercury in the operatory, and by removing a worn or broken amalgam restoration with a high-speed handpiece without water.

Mercury poisoning can cause birth defects, brain dysfunction, kidney problems, and other associated conditions. In addition, mercury poisoning is extremely dangerous because the dental team may never be aware that an office is contaminated until serious effects have taken place. The protocols for mercury hygiene should be an important consideration for the dental team. To prevent mercury poisoning, the following precautions should be taken:

1. Never touch amalgam or mercury with bare hands.
2. Enclose scrap amalgam in a tight container with used x-ray fixer or a specially prepared mercury solution that can be purchased from most supply companies (Figure 13-1). The solution in the container inactivates the mercury in the amalgam. A container specific for containment of scrap amalgam should be included in offices that use amalgam. Many states now require that dental offices install an amalgam separator. Such separators remove amalgam from waste water so less enters the sewage system. The amalgam in the separator and in the container needs to be collected and properly disposed of by a licensed professional company.
3. Try to prevent all mercury spills. If a spill does occur, special techniques should be followed. Always use one of the several devices that can be purchased for the purpose of collecting a spill. Never collect a mercury spill with the high-volume evacuation system or a vacuum cleaner.

4. When removing a worn or broken amalgam restoration, always use water with the high-speed handpiece. The high-volume evacuator suction tip should always be placed close to the operative site to catch any debris or dust removed from the tooth.
5. Most state governmental agencies have departments that will come into the dental office to monitor mercury levels upon request. This should be done on a routine basis.

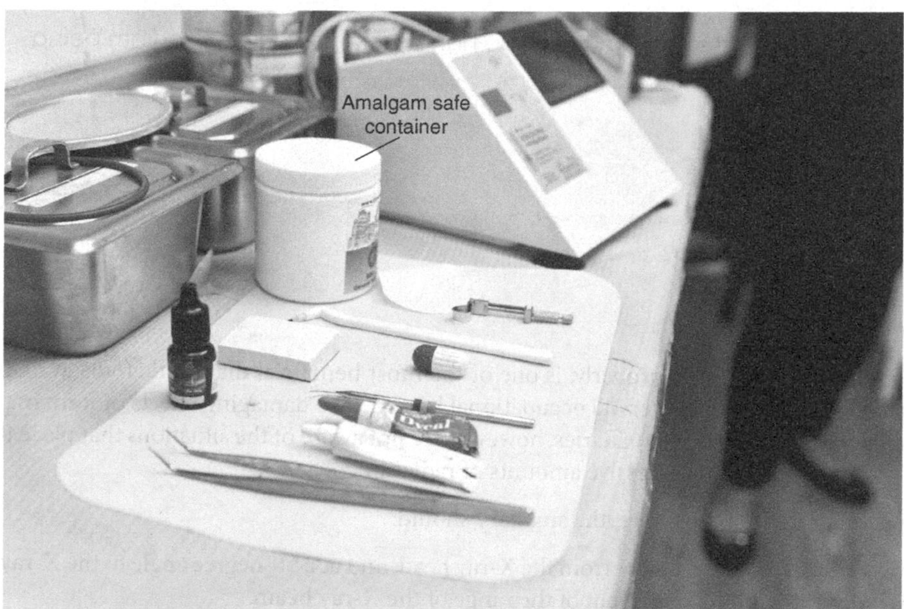

FIGURE 13-1 Amalgam container

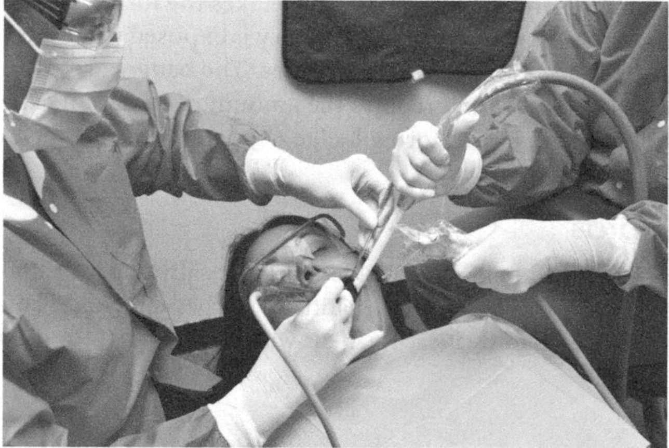

FIGURE 13-2 Use of high speed suction and water when removing existing amalgam

TEST YOUR KNOWLEDGE

1. How can the dental team reduce the chances of mercury contamination?

2. How should scrap amalgam be handled to prevent vapors from being released?

Radiation

Dental radiation, when used properly, is one of the most beneficial diagnostic tools available, but when used carelessly, it is a potential occupational hazard. The damaging effects of **ionizing radiation** are widely known. Some auxiliaries, however, are not aware of the situations that place them in danger of being exposed to excessive amounts of radiation.

To prevent radiation exposure, the auxiliary should:

1. Always be at least six feet away from the X-ray head, and at a 90-degree angle to the X-ray beam. This will place the technician out of the range of the X-ray beam.
2. If it is not possible to maintain a 6-foot distance, always stand behind a lead-lined shield to prevent any exposure to the ionizing radiation.
3. Never hold the image receptor in the patient's oral cavity.
4. Wear a personal monitoring device. This usually takes the form of a film badge that monitors the amounts of radiation to which an auxiliary is exposed (see Figure 13-3). These may be purchased through several different companies. The badges are returned each month to the company, which monitors and reports the amount of radiation exposure, if any. X-ray machines should also have a monitoring badge clipped to the outside exposure device.

Biological Hazards

The dental auxiliary is exposed to biological bloodborne or saliva-borne pathogens, ranging from human immunodeficiency virus (HIV) to hepatitis to herpes simplex. The standard of care in contemporary dental offices is to treat each patient with **universal precautions**, meaning that all

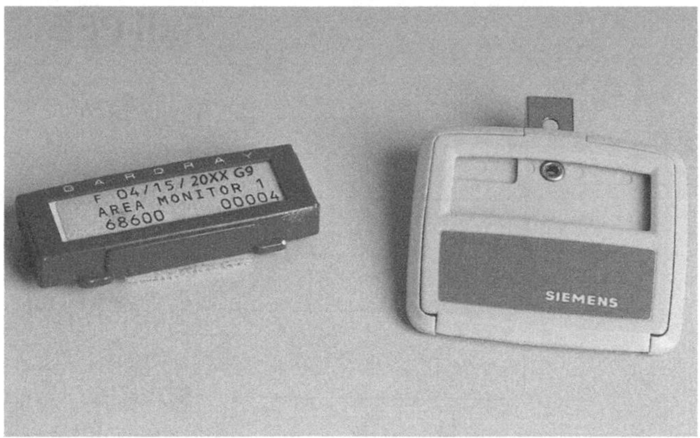

FIGURE 13-3 Monitoring badge for radiology machine and for operator

Source: Phinney/Halstead, Dental Assisting: A Comprehensive Approach 5e, Cengage, 2018.

patients are treated as if they are infectious. The hazard of exposure to biological pathogens is minimized by the use of **personal protective equipment (PPE)**. PPE should be worn for all procedures. PPE includes, but is not limited to, the following:

- Protective eyewear (i.e., goggles, dental face shield; see Figure 13-4)
- Gloves (i.e., latex, vinyl, etc.; see Figure 13-4)
- Masks (scc Figure 13-4)
- Protective clothing such as fluid repellant auxiliary gown or uniform (Figure 13-4)

Recently, with the COVID-19 pandemic, the Centers for Disease Control (CDC) stated that masks should be worn at all times in the dental office. During patient treatment, N95 respirator masks should be worn along with a face shield and hair covering. If aerosol generating procedures are scheduled, four handed dentistry with the use of high-speed suction should be implemented to minimize aerosols. Uniforms are not to be worn outside of the office. The dental health care worker should change into regular clothes when leaving the office and the uniform must be laundered by the dental office. The dental health care worker should be vaccinated against COVID-19 and should regularly check the CDC website for updates regarding infection control protocol. If there is a breakdown in the infection control standards, the auxiliary may be exposed to a biological hazard. In this situation, the dental auxiliary will need to follow the protocols mandated by the office, clinic, or institution that employs the auxiliary.

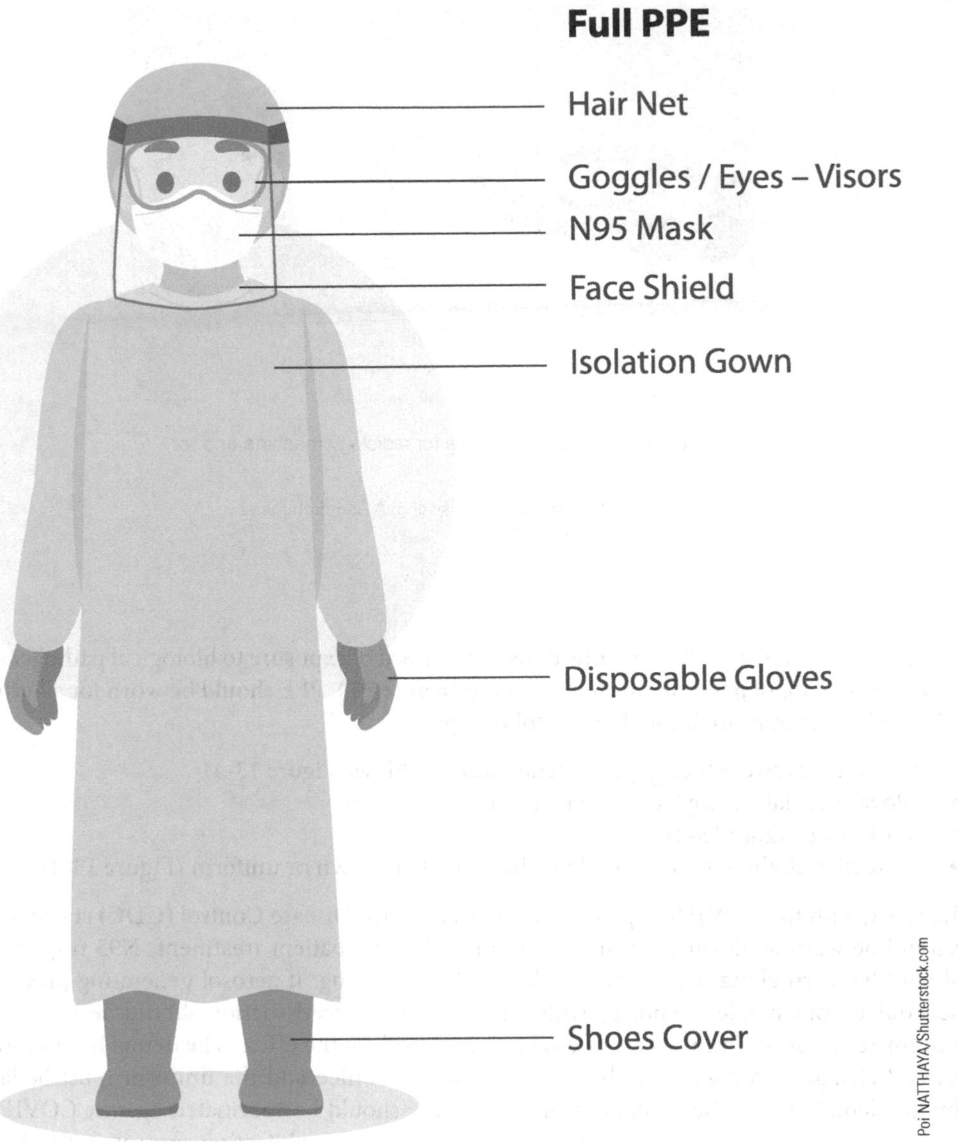

Full PPE

Hair Net

Goggles / Eyes – Visors

N95 Mask

Face Shield

Isolation Gown

Disposable Gloves

Shoes Cover

Poi NATHAYA/Shutterstock.com

FIGURE 13-4 Personal protective equipment

TEST YOUR KNOWLEDGE

1. When should the dental auxiliary hold a radiographic film in the patient's oral cavity?

2. What are some examples of PPE?

PATIENT DENTAL EMERGENCIES

This section describes some of the emergency situations that may occur in the office as a result of dental treatment. Many dentistry-related emergencies can occur, but this section is limited to those that seem to occur most often.

Broken Anesthetic Needle

An anesthetic needle may be broken during an injection because of poor technique by the dentist, a needle imperfection, or an abrupt violent movement by the patient. This kind of emergency occurs more often during a mandibular injection because of the position of the needle. The auxiliary can help prevent this emergency by examining the needle before the injection and by preventing the patient from grabbing or hitting the dentist's hand during the injection. Additionally, larger gauge (diameter) needs should be used as opposed to thinner finer needles, which are more prone to breakage.

If this emergency should occur, the patient should be informed of the situation by the dentist. The auxiliary should do everything possible to help keep the patient calm. Removal of a broken needle can be a complicated surgical procedure. Therefore, unless the dentist has extensive surgical experience, the patient is usually referred to an oral surgeon. The auxiliary should record the entire incident in the patient's chart. This may prove valuable should later legal action be taken.

Separated Endodontic Reamer or File

During endodontic therapy, an **endodontic file** or **reamer** (Figure 13-5) may separate and remain in the root canal of the tooth (Figure 13-6). In some cases, it may not be possible to remove the file and it will then remain in the tooth. The patient should be made aware of this and the tooth should be monitored. The auxiliary must be prepared to assist with any procedure the dentist chooses.

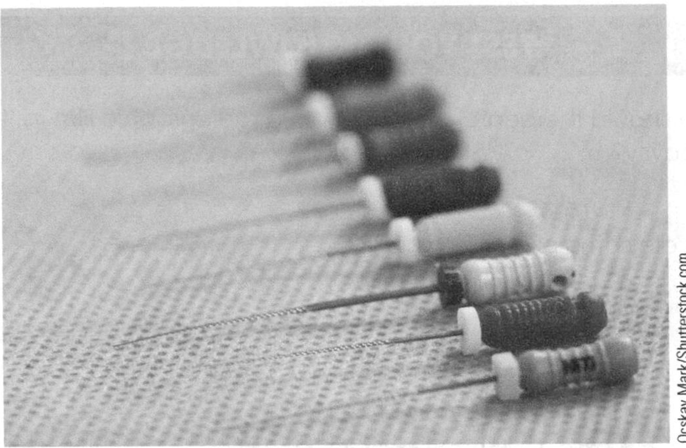

FIGURE 13-5 Root canal files

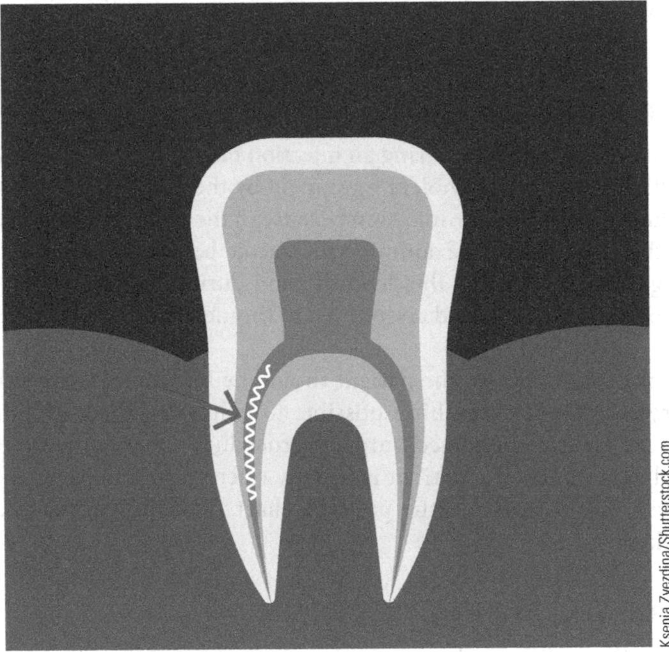

FIGURE 13-6 Drawing of a broken file in the tooth canal

Soft-Tissue Injury

During surgical procedures, it is extremely common for the surgical site to become slippery, and consequently it is easy for a sharp surgical instrument to slip off the tooth and lacerate the surrounding soft tissues. This may wound the tongue, cheek, or gingival areas. The dentist will treat each such area as required, and the auxiliary should be prepared to assist with any necessary procedure.

In some situations, the auxiliary can help to prevent laceration of the soft tissue by providing proficient suctioning, which keeps the area clear and increases visibility. The auxiliary also can use a mirror or other instrument to retract the oral soft tissues and tongue from the operative field.

TEST YOUR KNOWLEDGE

1. How can the dental auxiliary prevent an anesthetic needle from breaking?
2. Why is there potential for soft tissue injury present during dental procedures?

Nitrous Oxide/Oxygen Conscious Sedation

Nitrous oxide/oxygen conscious sedation is being used with increasing frequency in today's dental office. When used properly, it provides a more pleasant experience for most anxious dental patients due to its **anxiolytic** properties. On the other hand, if used incorrectly, nitrous oxide/oxygen conscious sedation can become a hazard not only to the patient but also to the dental team.

During recent years, it has become known that continuous exposure to nitrous oxide/oxygen vapors can be hazardous to dental personnel. When nitrous oxide/oxygen conscious sedation is administered through a nosepiece, traces of the gas can leak around the nasal hood. In the past, the dental team was constantly inhaling these escaping vapors. Physical problems such as miscarriages and infertility have been noted to occur as a result of this exposure. Today's units have an attachment (known as a scavenger unit) that eliminates any trace gas. All units are required to have this attachment.

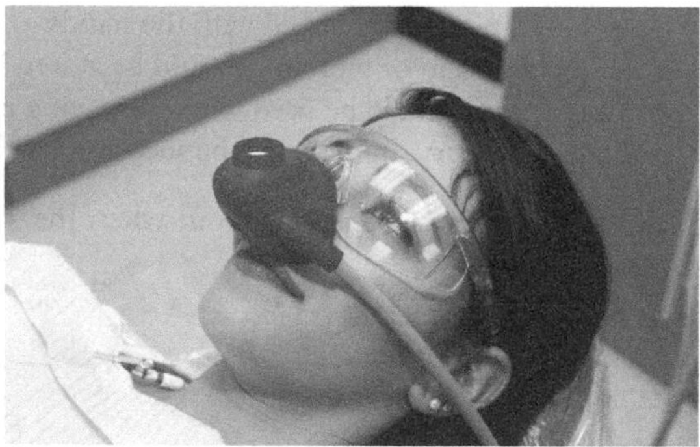

FIGURE 13-7 Nitrous oxide sedation with nasal hood

Source: Phinney/Halstead, Dental Assisting: A Comprehensive Approach 5e, Cengage, 2018.

When administered at the proper dose and rate, nitrous oxide/oxygen conscious sedation provides a good sedative for the dental patient. However, if the dose is high, the substance functions as a general anesthetic and the patient may lose consciousness, presenting a serious condition in the dental office that should always be avoided.

To achieve optimal effects from nitrous oxide/oxygen conscious sedation, the dental team must properly explain its effects to the patient. The gas should then be introduced through **titration**. The dental team should communicate with the patient regarding the signs and symptoms of the effects of nitrous oxide. These include tingling in the extremities, a feeling of warmth, and a feeling of relaxation. Oversedation can lead to excitement and hallucinations, nausea, and vomiting. This results in a negative experience with nitrous oxide. This is usually due to operator error resulting in oversedation. Nitrous oxide/oxygen conscious sedation, when administered and monitored properly, can be used safely and effectively. However, the auxiliary should be aware that there are potential complications associated with the use of this form of sedation.

SUMMARY

The dental office can present both the dental team and the patient with hazardous situations. The auxiliary should realize that most of these situations may be prevented if proper precautions are taken. However, no matter what prevention techniques are employed, some emergencies will occur. It is these situations that the auxiliary needs to know how to handle properly.

REVIEW QUESTIONS

MULTIPLE CHOICE

1. Which of the following is not true concerning the handling of mercury?
   a. It should never be touched with the hands.
   b. Scrap amalgam or mercury should be stored in a dry container.
   c. Water spray should be used when removing an old amalgam.
   d. Excess mercury should never be suctioned with the high-volume suction.

2. If the auxiliary must be in the room when the x-ray is being exposed, the auxillary should be
   a. at the patient's feet.
   b. behind a lead screen.
   c. holding the tube head.
   d. all the above

3. The auxiliary may prevent the breaking of an anesthetic needle by
   a. using a larger-gauge needle.
   b. keeping the patient from hitting the dentist's hands.

c. inspecting the needle before use.
d. all the above

4. Which of the following are necessary for optimum protection from infectious diseases?
   a. mask
   b. gloves
   c. safety glasses
   d. all the above

5. To eliminate constant exposure to nitrous oxide/oxygen vapors, the dental team should use a unit that has which of the following?
   a. scavenger unit
   b. full face mask
   c. clear nasal hood
   d. none of the above

6. Which of the following is correct regarding the hazards of mercury?
   a. Scrap amalgam can be stored in any dry container.
   b. Mercury can be absorbed through the skin.
   c. Scrap amalgam can be thrown out with the regular trash.
   d. Water is not required when removing existing amalgam from a tooth.

7. Which of the following is correct regarding ionizing radiation?
   a. Ionizing radiation is harmless.
   b. It is acceptable for the operator to hold the image receptor in position while exposing radiographs.
   c. The operator should wear a personal monitoring device for exposure to ionizing radiation.
   d. The operator should stand at a 20 degree angle to the X-ray beam.

8. Local anesthetic needles may break if the patient suddenly moves during the injection. Breakage is most likely to occur with mandibular injections.
   a. Both statements are true.
   b. Both statements are false.
   c. The first statement is true, the second statement is false.
   d. The first statement is false, the second statement is true.

9. Endodontic instruments may break in the canal during treatment. There is no need to advise the patient about this occurrence.
   a. Both statements are true.
   b. Both statements are false.
   c. The first statement is true, the second statement is false.
   d. The first statement is false, the second statement is true.

10. Which of the following is not correct regarding nitrous oxide sedation?
    a. Nitrous oxide is beneficial because it has anxiolytic properties.
    b. Nitrous oxide equipment should have scavenging capabilities.
    c. Oversedation with nitrous oxide leads to a pleasant patient experience.
    d. Optimal sedation symptoms include tingling of the extremities.

TRUE OR FALSE

_______ 1. Broken anesthetic needles occur most often during maxillary injections.

_______ 2. A broken endodontic file may not need to be removed from the canal.

_______ 3. For optimal benefits, nitrous oxide should be titrated when administered.

_______ 4. A scavenger unit is not needed on today's nitrous oxide/oxygen conscious sedation units.

_______ 5. It is acceptable to clean up spilled mercury with bare hands.

_______ 6. In the dental office, mercury exposure usually occurs through inhalation of improperly stored scrap amalgam.

_______ 7. It is not necessary to use high-speed suction when removing an existing amalgam from a patient's tooth.

_______ 8. The operator should stand in the path of the X-ray beam when exposing patient radiographs.

_______ 9. There is no need to wear full PPE while exposing radiographs since no aerosols are being generated.

_______ 10. Soft tissue injuries can be prevented by suctioning the operative field and retracting soft tissues in the area.

MEDICAL EMERGENCY!

CASE STUDY 13-1

A 35-year-old female presents with a negative medical history. The treatment plan for today is to have a crown placed on tooth number 3. The patient is anxious and requests nitrous oxide sedation. Since this was not previously planned, time is a little short so the nitrous is administered quickly. Shortly thereafter, the patient starts to feel nauseous.

Questions

1. Why did the patient start to feel nauseous?
2. What should have been done differently to avoid this problem?
3. What should be done for future appointments in terms of scheduling?

CASE STUDY 13-2

A 48-year-old male presents with a negative medical history. The treatment plan for today's appointment is to complete an endodontic procedure on tooth number 14. As treatment progresses, a small portion of an endodontic file breaks off in the canal of the tooth.

Questions

1. How should this situation be handled to reduce the risk to the patient and dental team?

CHAPTER 14

Legalities of Emergency Care

LEARNING OUTCOMES

Upon completion of this chapter, the student will be able to:

- Explain the dental team's general legal duties to the patient
- Explain the Good Samaritan law
- Explain the ways a dental team can prevent lawsuits against them

KEY TERMS

abandonment
negligence

This chapter is designed to provide the dental auxiliary with basic information concerning legal problems associated with emergency care. Laws vary from state to state, and auxiliaries should check the laws pertaining to the state of their employment. Furthermore, laws that could affect the outcome of a particular legal action are changing every day, so it is important to stay up-to-date in this area.

DUTIES AND RESPONSIBILITIES

The number of lawsuits against health professionals is growing. To reduce the risk of such a case, the dental team must first understand its legal obligations to the patient. A failure of the dental team to meet any of its legal duties leaves the team liable for a lawsuit based mainly on **negligence**. See emergency basics box 14-1 for a summary of the duties and responsibilities.

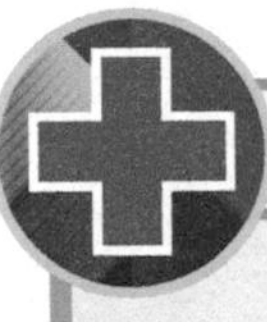

Emergency Basics 14-1

Duties and Responsibilities

Duty to Treat
Duty Not to Abandon
Duty of Preparedness

Duty to Treat

The dental team has an obligation, once a patient has been accepted for care, to provide all the treatment required by the patient. In an emergency, the dental team must do everything in its power to provide care for the patient. This treatment requirement also includes the transfer of the patient to a hospital if the scope of the emergency requires more extensive care than that available in the dental office. In most cases the dentist or dental team does not cause the medical emergency. As a result, the dentist would not be found liable for the medical emergency. However, if the dental team does not manage the emergency properly, the dentist would be held liable. For example, if a patient has a history of heart disease and suffered a myocardial infarction in the chair, the dentist would not be at fault for the infarction. However, if the dentist did not provide an aspirin to the patient to chew while waiting for Emergency Medical Services (EMS) or did not provide oxygen while waiting for EMS and the patient died, the dentist may be held liable for poor management.

Duty Not to Abandon

Once the dental team begins to treat the patient, they has a duty not to abandon the patient. In an emergency situation, this means the dentist must first stabilize the patient, implement appropriate steps in managing the emergency, and then transfer the patient to a medical facility if necessary. If the dental team did not initiate emergency management on the patient but merely summoned transportation to a medical facility, the patient may have grounds for legal action. Furthermore, the dental team must never allow the patient to leave the dental office until the emergency is over. For example, if a patient complains of chest pain, is allowed by the dental team to leave while still experiencing the pain, and subsequently experiences a myocardial infarction, it is extremely possible that the patient can sue the dental team for negligence on the grounds of **abandonment**.

Duty of Preparedness

The dental team has a legal duty to the patient to be prepared for an emergency. First, the dental team must have the knowledge to administer basic care in the event of an emergency. Second, the office must contain basic emergency equipment such as an oxygen tank and a complete emergency kit. Third, the dentist and staff must be trained in basic emergency management as well as CPR/BLS.

The dentist is ultimately responsible for the actions of employees while they are at work. However, dental auxiliaries can still be held liable for their actions and included in any lawsuit against the dentist. Auxiliaries therefore have the legal obligation to be prepared for an emergency by being trained in emergency treatment such as CPR.

GOOD SAMARITAN LAW

Most states have enacted Good Samaritan laws. These laws, which give legal protection to people who provide emergency care to ill or injured people, have been developed to encourage people to help others in emergency situations. They require that the "Good Samaritan" use common sense and a reasonable level of skill, and not exceed the scope of the individual's training in emergency situations. They assume that people will do their best to save a life or prevent further injury.

People are rarely sued for helping in an emergency. However, the existence of Good Samaritan laws does not mean that someone cannot be sued in that situation. In rare court cases, courts have ruled that these laws did not apply where an individual rescuer's actions were grossly or willfully negligent or reckless or where the rescuer abandoned the victim after initiating care.

Dental office staff should always be current in their CPR and emergency training and be prepared to assist a patient in the event of an emergency.

TEST YOUR KNOWLEDGE

1. Which member of the dental team is ultimately responsible for the actions of the entire dental team?

2. Can a dental team be liable for not completing emergency management for a patient? Why or why not?

PREVENTING LEGAL PROBLEMS

The dental team cannot prevent every medical emergency. Similarly, the dental team cannot prevent a patient from bringing legal action. However, the dental team can do several things to prevent the patient from being successful if there is litigation.

First, the dental team must do everything possible to prevent an emergency from occurring. This can be achieved by utilizing optimum dental techniques such as optimum pain management and stress reduction protocol; by maintaining updated medical histories; obtaining medical consults when warranted; being current in CPR/BLS; and by having the necessary knowledge and equipment to handle an emergency.

Second, the dental team should establish an emergency routine and practice it on a regular basis. This demonstrates that the team is prepared and also enables the team to act more efficiently and effectively during an emergency.

Third, the dental office should have all emergency numbers available near the phone. One office member should be designated to summon medical assistance when needed.

Finally, should an emergency occur, the auxiliary should write down, in detail, everything that transpired prior to, during, and after the emergency. This will prove extremely important if a patient sues, enabling the defense to present the court with the pertinent facts of the emergency.

SUMMARY

Patients can initiate lawsuits against any member of the dental team. Each state's legal requirements for the dental team differ. It is important for the dental team to be aware of its responsibilities. By being aware of those responsibilities, the dental team will be better prepared to prevent legal actions or to answer them.

REVIEW QUESTIONS

MULTIPLE CHOICE

1. Which law gives legal protection to people who provide emergency care to ill or injured people?
   a. ADAA Code of Ethics
   b. Americans with Disabilities Act
   c. Good Samaritan Law
   d. HIPAA

2. Which of the following is not a general legal duty to the patient?
   a. not to abandon
   b. preparedness

c. treat
d. all of the above are general legal duties to the patient

3. A patient experiencing documented numbness caused by a transient ischemic attack is allowed to leave the dental office still exhibiting numbness. The patient later experiences a cerebrovascular accident. The patient can sue the dental team based on what grounds of legal duty?
   a. abandonment
   b. ethics
   c. preparedness
   d. none of the above

4. Which of the following is/are necessary to fulfill the legal duty of preparedness in a dental office?
   a. basic emergency equipment
   b. knowledge to administer basic life support
   c. training in basic emergency treatment
   d. all of the above

5. Who is ultimately responsible for the actions that occur in the dental office?
   a. dental office manager
   b. dental auxiliary
   c. dentist
   d. receptionist

TRUE/FALSE

_______ 1. The dental staff does not have to have current CPR and emergency training.

_______ 2. A failure of a dental team to meet any of its legal duties leaves the team liable for a lawsuit.

_______ 3. The laws pertaining to emergency treatment are the same in each state.

_______ 4. Negligence occurs if the dental team fails to meet any of its legal duties.

_______ 5. Good Samaritan laws help to prevent the person who received emergency care from suing the person who provided the emergency care.

MEDICAL EMERGENCY!

CASE STUDY 14-1

A 45-year-old female presents with a negative medical history. She has come to the dental office for a checkup and cleaning. During the appointment, the patient experiences chest pains. The dental team determines that the patient is possibly experiencing a myocardial infarction. They provide emergency management for the patient and call for emergency medical assistance. The oxygen tank is empty and they are not able to provide oxygen to the patient. They also do not have aspirin in the emergency kit. The patient is transported to the hospital.

Questions

1. What was done wrong?

2. Can the patient sue?

3. What should be done to avoid such problems in the future?

Glossary

A

abandonment Form of malpractice that occurs when a health care provider ends a provider/patient relationship without notice that is reasonable or without allowing the patient to find an alternate caregiver.
absence (petit mal) seizure An epileptic seizure characterized by a sudden momentary loss of consciousness occasionally accompanied by minor twitching
acetylcholine A neurotransmitter of the parasympathetic nervous system
albuterol Bronchodilating agent that is used to manage asthma
alkalosis An abnormal increase in the alkalinity of the blood
allergen Any substance capable of inducing an allergic reaction
allergic Reaction of an immune system to a substance
American Society of Anesthesiologists (ASA) Research and scientific physician's association
ammonia Has formula NH_3 and a pungent odor
ampule Sealed gas capsule which usually contains a liquid
amyl nitrite A vasodilator
anaphylactic Serious allergic reaction which can be life threatening
anaphylaxis A severe life-threatening allergic reaction
aneurysm Abnormality of a blood vessel, usually an artery, caused most often by a defect or weakness of the vessel wall
angina pectoris A severe pain in and around the heart caused by an insufficient supply of oxygenated blood to the heart
angina Chest pain caused by reduced blood flow to the heart muscle
angioedema An allergic reaction characterized by swelling of the skin or mucous membrane
antecubital fossa Area approximately one inch from the elbow at which the stethoscope is placed to hear the pulse when measuring blood pressure
antibody A protein produced to react specifically with an antigen
anticoagulant Preventing the change of blood from liquid to solid
antigen Substance that causes the formation of an antibody; also known as *allergen*
antihypertensive Drugs used to treat hypertension
anxiolytic An agent that breaks up anxiety
aorta Main artery of the human body
aphasia Difficulty in speaking
arrhythmia Abnormal heart rate
arteriosclerosis Thickening of the artery walls that results in loss of elasticity
arteriosclerotic Thickening of the vessel walls
ASA Physical Status Classification System (ASAPSCS) System to assess a patient's pre-anesthesia risk for a medical emergency
asphyxiation Death caused by lack of oxygen
aspirate To breathe in forcefully causing an object to become lodged in the airway
assessment Evaluation
ataxia A loss in the coordination of the muscles
atherosclerosis Form of arteriosclerosis that affects the coronary arteries and causes coronary artery disease

atria Upper chambers of the heart

atrial fibrillation Rapid irregular muscle contractions of the heart causing an irregular rhythm

atrioventricular valve A valve in the heart through which blood flows from the atria to the ventricles

aura A sight, sound, or smell unique to an individual before experiencing an epileptic seizure

B

baseline vital signs Vital signs (e.g., blood pressure, pulse, respiration rate, and temperature) that are recorded prior to treatment to help determine how the patient is responding during treatment.

biofilm A collection of microorganisms such as bacteria and fungi that grow on oral surfaces

blood pressure The pressure the blood exerts on the walls of the arteries, the veins, and the chambers of the heart

bradypnea Slow breathing rate

bronchioles A smaller branch of the bronchus

bronchodilators Medications that dilate the airways and are used to treat asthma

C

carbon dioxide A colorless, odorless gas produced by the oxidation of carbon

cardiac arrhythmias Abnormal rhythms of the heart

carotid artery Artery located on either side of the neck; used to measure the pulse during an emergency

cerebrovascular accident A lack of blood flow to the brain caused by a sudden rupture or blockage

clonic Movements marked by contraction and relaxation of muscles that are associated with a tonic-clonic (grand mal) seizure

congestive heart failure Condition in which the heart is failing as a pump

contact dermatitis Inflammation of the skin from contact with a sensitizing agent

convulsion A violent and sudden and unusual movement of the body that is a result of involuntary muscle contractions

coronary artery disease A condition in which the walls of the coronary arteries become thick and hard

cricothyrotomy Incision made through the skin and the cricothyroid ligament to establish a temporary airway

cyanosis Lack of oxygen in the blood causing blueness in the skin

D

demand-valve resuscitator used to ventilate a patient that has stopped breathing

demographic Related to a population

dental dam A thin sheet of latex or nonlatex rubber for isolating one or more teeth during a dental procedure

diabetic coma Loss of consciousness related to severely elevated blood sugar

diastolic blood pressure Pressure on the arteries when the heart relaxes between beats

diazepam A medication used to treat active seizures; also used to treat anxiety, nervousness, and muscle spasms

Dilantin gingival hyperplasia Overgrowth of gingival tissue that results from the intake of Dilantin.

diuretic Drugs that increase the passing out of urine

Down syndrome Genetic disorder caused by a third chromosome 21, also called trisomy 21

dysphagia Difficulty in swallowing

E

edema Local or generalized swelling from retention of excessive fluid

electrolyte Essential minerals

embolism A clot that forms somewhere in the body and travels throughout the body until it lodges in a smaller vessel

emergency kit Contains essential medications and supplies yo respond to more common medical emergencies

endocardium Lining of the inner heart surface
endodontic file Instrument used in root canal therapy
endodontic reamer Instrument used in root canal therapy
engulf Special cells that enfolds around foreign particle and swallow it up; important bodily defense against infection
epicardium Inner layer of the pericardium
epigastrium Area of the upper abdomen
epilepsy A type of seizure disorder that affects people for a variety of reasons and is not selective as to ethnicity, age, or gender
epileptic cry A short, loud cry that results from a sudden contraction of the chest, causing the air to rush out of the lungs
epinephrine Vasoconstrictor and bronchodilator
erythema Redness of the skin
extrinsic asthma A form of asthma caused by the exposure of the bronchial mucosa to an inhaled airborne antigen

F

febrile Having a fever
fibrin An elastic protein that forms from fibrinogen when blood clots
flowmeter Used to measure a volume of gas

G

gestational diabetes Diabetes that occurs during pregnancy and usually resolves after childbirth
gingival hyperplasia Overgrowth of the gingival tissue around the teeth
glucagon Hormone produced by pancreas that works to raise blood glucose
glucose Simple sugar that is the main type found in blood

H

HbA1C Test to measure the amount of sugar bound to hemoglobin in red blood cells
Health Insurance Portability and Accountability Act (HIPAA) Federal law that set national standards to protect personal health information
Heimlich maneuver Technique used to remove an object that is lodged in the airway
hemiparalysis Paralysis or muscle weakness on one side of the body that affects arms, legs, facial muscles
hemiplegia Paralysis of one side of the body
hemorrhagic A large amount of blood loss in a short period of time
histamine Substance normally found in the body; its functions include increasing gastric secretions, constriction of the smooth muscles of the bronchioles, and dilation of capillaries
histamine Agent released by cells in response to injury or to an allergy
hyperglycemia Elevated blood sugar
hypertension Abnormally high pressure of the blood against the arterial walls
hypocarbia A decrease in the carbon dioxide in the blood
hypoglycemia Low blood sugar
hypoxia Condition of oxygen deprivation in part or all of the body

I

idiopathic A disease or condition that is from an unknown cause
immune system A biological complex that protects the body against pathogenic organisms and other foreign bodies
immunoglobulin system Five structurally and antigenically distinct antibodies present in the serum and external secretions of the body
insulin Hormone produced by the islets of Langerhan cells in the pancreas that functions to regulate blood sugar
insulin shock Also known as hypoglycemia or low blood sugar
interferons Proteins produced by cells in response to a virus to block viral replication

intracerebral Existing within the cerebrum
intrinsic asthma A nonallergic form of asthma usually first occurring later in life that tends to be chronic and persistent rather than episodic
ionizing radiation X-rays that have the ability to cause the removal of an electron from an atom or a molecule
ischemia Inadequate blood supply to an organ or part of the body
ischemic Deficiency of blood supply

J

Jacksonian seizure A simple partial (focal or localized) seizure

K

ketones Produced when cells need energy and the body burns fat for fuel
Korotkoff sounds Arterial sounds heard through a stethoscope used to determine systolic and diastolic blood pressure while using a sphygmomanometer cuff

L

latex allergy A medical term encompassing a range of allergic reactions to natural rubber latex
lumen The cavity of a tubular organ such as a blood vessel
lymphocytes Clear thin fluid that circulates through the body and collects bacteria

M

macrovascular disease Disease of large vessels in the body such as the aorta
magnetic resonance image Scan that uses powerful magnets to create an image of a body area
medical history Information gained by healthcare provider by asking specific questions related to health
microvascular disease Disease of small vessels in the body
myocardial infarction Heart attack
myocardium Middle layer of the heart wall

N

naloxone Reversal agent used in the event of a narcotic overdose
nasal cannula Device which delivers supplemental oxygen
negligence Improper care of a patient that results in a malpractice claim by the patient.
neoprene Synthetic rubber resistant to oils, water, and solvents
neuropathy Weakness, pain, or a numbing sensation usually caused by nerve damage, most common in the feet and the hands
nitroglycerine Vasodilator used to manage angina
nonpsychogenic Physical, nonpsychological causes of a condition
nosocomial Disease that originates in a hospital or health care setting

O

opioid Class of drugs used to reduce pain
oral hypoglycemic Oral medications to lower blood sugar
orthostatic hypotension Decrease in blood pressure when a person is raised supine to erect
oxygen mask Device used to deliver oxygen
oxygen tank Cylinder which contains oxygen

P

palliative Relieving symptoms without curing
pancreas Organ that produces several hormones including insulin
partial (focal or localized) seizure Convulsive movements associated with epilepsy occurring on one side of the body only
pericardium Sac that encloses the heart
periodontal disease Infection of the soft tissues that hold the teeth in place
perioral Around the oral cavity

personal protective equipment (PPE) Equipment including but not limited to protective eyewear, gloves, masks, protective clothing
phagocytes Cell that engulfs and destroys invaders such as bacteria and viruses
Physician's Desk Reference (PDR) Provides prescribing information related to prescription medications
platelet A cell involved in the clotting of the blood
polydipsia Excess thirst
polyphagia Extreme hunger
polyuria Frequent urination
postural hypotension Also called orthostatic hypotension; abnormal drop in blood pressure upon assuming the upright position, which may lead to loss of consciousness
presyncope First stage of syncope; stage prior to the actual loss of consciousness
prodromal Signs or symptoms that mark the onset of a disease
protected health information (PHI) Information related to payment for medical services, health history, treatment or diagnosis that is protected from disclosure under federal law
psychogenic Psychological causes of a condition
pulmonary artery Artery that runs from the right ventricle to the lungs
pulse The regular expansion and contraction of an artery caused by the ejection of the blood from the left ventricle of the heart as it contracts

R

radial artery An artery located in the forearm
regulator Valve that controls the pressure of a gas or liquid in a cylinder or tank
respiration rate The number of times that a person inhales and exhales

S

semilunar valves Valves with half-moon-shaped cusps, for example, the aortic valve and the pulmonary valve
shock A life-threatening condition that occurs when the body is not getting enough blood flow
sickle cell anemia An inherited blood disorder where the red blood cells change to a sickle shape, causing them to die off earlier
sildenafil Vasodilator used to treat erectile dysfunction
sodium hypochlorite An endodontic antimicrobial irrigant
sphygmomanometer Instrument that consists of a gauge and an inflatable bag inside an armband; used to measure blood pressure
status asthmaticus A severe form of asthma in which the victim experiences a continuous asthma attack
status epilepticus Situation in which a person experiences one seizure after another or one continuous seizure
stethoscope Instrument used to listen to the heart and chest sounds
stridor A severe vibrating sound
subarachnoid Situated below the arachnoid membrane, a web-like membrane that covers the brain and spinal cord
subcutaneous Applied under the skin
substernal Behind the sternum
supine position Lying horizontally on the back with knees and nose in the same plane
sympathetic autonomic nervous system Involuntary autonomic nervous system that increases blood flow to the heart and increases heart rate, causes pupil dilation
systolic blood pressure Pressure on the arteries when the heart is beating, or working

T

tachycardia Fast resting heart rate
tachypnea Rapid breathing rate
tadalafil Vasodilator used to treat erectile dysfunction
temperature The level of heat in the body
thrombosis A clot that forms in a vessel

titration Administration of a drug in small increments either through inhalation or intravenous methods until the desired level of effect is obtained
tonic Movements characterized by continuous tension or contraction of muscles that are associated with a tonic-clonic (grand mal) seizure
tonic-clonic (grand mal) seizure An epileptic seizure characterized by generalized involuntary muscular contraction and cessation of respiration followed by tonic and clonic spasms of the muscles
trachea The air passage that descends from the larynx and branches into the right and left bronchi; also known as the *windpipe*
tracheobronchial tree The trachea, bronchi, and the bronchial tubes
tracheostomy Incision made through the skin into the trachea to relieve an airway obstruction
Trendelenburg position Position in which the patient is supine with the feet higher than the head
tricyclic antidepressants A class of medications that is used to treat depression

U

universal precautions Infection control practices that apply to patient treatment regardless of patient health status. These practices help to prevent the spread of diseases.
urticaria A skin reaction characterized by the eruption of itching wheals; also known as *hives*

V

vaporole Small capsule which contains a volatile drug
vasodilator An agent that causes the dilation of blood vessels
vasodilator Medications that dilate blood vessels
vasovagal syncope Also referred to as vasodepressor syncope; loss of consciousness that results from overactivity of the vagus nerve, which causes bradycardia and hypotension
ventricles Lower chambers of the heart
verdanafil Vasodilator used to treat erectile dysfunction
vesicle An elevation of the epidermis containing fluid; also known as a *blister*

W

warfarin Common anticoagulant medication

References

Publications

Eisenberg, M. S., & Mengert, T. J. (2001). Cardiac resuscitation. *New England Journal of Medicine, 344*, 1304–1313. https://www.nejm.org/doi/full/10.1056/NEJM200104263441707

Haas, D. A. (2010). Preparing dental office staff members for emergencies: Developing a basic action plan. *Journal of the American Dental Association, 141*(1), S8–S13. https://doi.org/10.14219/jada.archive.2010.0352

Haveles, E. B. (2019). Applied pharmacology for the dental hygienist (8th ed.). St. Louis, MO: Elsevier.

Little, J. W., Falace, D. Q., Miller, C. S., & Rhodus, N. L. (2017). *Dental management of the medically compromised patient* (6th ed.). Elsevier Health Sciences.

Malamed, S. F. (2007). *Medical emergencies in the dental office* (7th ed.). Elsevier Health Sciences.

Malamed, S., 2010. Knowing Your Patients. *The Journal of the American Dental Association*, 141, pp. S3–S7.

Phinney, D. J., & Halstead, J. H. (2018). *Dental assisting: A comprehensive approach* (5th ed.). Thomson Learning/Delmar.

Pickett, F., & Guerenlian, J. (2005). *The medical history: Clinical implications and emergency prevention in dental settings.* Lippincott Williams & Wilkins.

Wilkins, E. M. (2020). *Clinical practice of the dental hygienist* (13th ed.). Lippincott Williams & Wilkins.

Internet Resources

American Dental Association. (n.d.). http://www.ada.org

American Diabetes Association. (n.d.). http://www.diabetes.org

American Heart Association. (2021). https://www.heart.org/

American Heart Association. (2020). *2020 American Heart Association Guidelines for CPR and ECC.* https://cpr.heart.org/en/resuscitation-science/cpr-and-ecc-guidelines

American Lung Association. (n.d.). https://www.lung.org/

American Red Cross. (n.d.). http://www.redcross.org

American Stroke Association. (2021). https://www.stroke.org/

Asthma and Allergy Foundation of America. (2021). *Asthma.* https://www.aafa.org/

Cleveland Clinic for Continuing Education. (2021). Disease management: https://www.clevelandclinicmeded.com/medicalpubs/diseasemanagement/cardiology/

Epilepsy Foundation. (n.d.). https://www.epilepsy.com/

Health and Human Serivces. (2013). *Summary of the HIPAA Security Rule.* https://www.hhs.gov/hipaa/for-professionals/security/laws-regulations/index.html

HealthFirst. (2019). *Guidelines for Emergency Medical Kits for Dental Offices.* https://www.healthfirst.com/blog/guidelines-for-emergency-medical-kits-for-dental-offices/

The Free Dictionary. (2021). *Medical dictionary.* Farlex. http://medical-dictionary.thefreedictionary.com

Mayo Clinic. (2021). Diabetic ketoacidosis. http://www.mayoclinic.com/health/diabetic-ketoacidosis/DS00674/DSECTION=symptoms

Mayo Clinic. (2021). Hypothyroidism (underactive thyroid). http://www.mayoclinic.com/health/hypothyroidism/DS00353/DSECTION=symptoms

Mayo Clinic. (2021). *Low blood pressure.* http://www.mayoclinic.com/health/low-blood-pressure/DS00590/DSECTION=causes

Medscape. (2020). Cardiogenic pulmonary edema. http://emedicine.medscape.com/article/157452-overview

Merriam-Webster. (2021). The Merriam-Webster.com Dictionary. https://www.merriam-webster.com/

National Heart, Lung, and Blood Institute. (2020). *Asthma.* https://www.nhlbi.nih.gov/health-topics/asthma

National Heart, Lung, and Blood Institute. (n.d.). *COPD.* https://www.nhlbi.nih.gov/health-topics/copd

OSHA. (2013). *First Aid and Patient Emergency Kits in the Dental Office.* https://osha review.com/2013/01/first-aid-and-patient-emergency-kits-in-the-dental-office/

Index

A

B

C

D

E

F

G

H

I

J

K

L

M

N

O

P

Q

R

S

T

U

V

W

X